# Mentoring and Supervision in Healthcare

SAGE has been part of the global academic community since 1965, supporting high quality research and learning that transforms society and our understanding of individuals, groups, and cultures. SAGE is the independent, innovative, natural home for authors, editors and societies who share our commitment and passion for the social sciences.

Find out more at: **www.sagepublications.com**

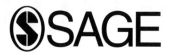

2nd edition

# Mentoring and Supervision in Healthcare

## Neil Gopee

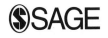

Los Angeles | London | New Delhi
Singapore | Washington DC

This edition first published 2011
First edition published 2008

SAGE Publications Ltd
1 Oliver's Yard
55 City Road
London EC1Y 1SP

SAGE Publications Inc.
2455 Teller Road
Thousand Oaks, California 91320

SAGE Publications India Pvt Ltd
B 1/I 1 Mohan Cooperative Industrial Area
Mathura Road
New Delhi 110 044

SAGE Publications Asia-Pacific Pte Ltd
33 Pekin Street #02-01
Far East Square
Singapore 048763


**Library of Congress Control Number: 2010939005**

**British Library Cataloguing in Publication data**

A catalogue record for this book is available from the British Library

ISBN 978-0-85702-418-3
ISBN 978-0-85702-419-0 (pbk)




Typeset by C&M Digitals (P) Ltd, Chennai, India
Printed by CPI Antony Rowe, Chippenham, Wiltshire
Printed on paper from sustainable resources

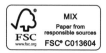

# Contents

# List of Boxes, Figures and Tables

## Boxes

# Figures

# Tables

# About the Author

I am currently employed as a Senior Lecturer in Health and Life Sciences at Coventry University, and have until very recently also worked as Associate Lecturer for the Open University. My role as external examiner at various Higher Education Institutions in my subject areas has also broadened my insights into the two subject areas that I teach and research: (1) learning, teaching and assessment (under- and post-graduate), and (2) management and leadership in healthcare settings.

I qualified as a nurse in the 1970s and worked in general surgical nursing for a year before moving on to complete the 'registered mental health nurse' course. Through my nursing career, a combination of clinical experiences in primary care and general intensive care nursing was also supplemented by attendance at numerous professional development short and long courses, including various workshops on writing for publication and completing my doctorate in continuing professional education at Warwick University.

My first peer-reviewed article was published in 1991 based on my then nurse tutor role. The 1990s were when nurse education programmes became a part of university provision, which further opened up authoring opportunities, and I negotiated with Alison Poyner, Commissioning Editor at SAGE publications, to write the *Mentoring and Supervision in Healthcare* book, the first edition of which was published in 2007. Along the way, I also worked with SAGE publications to write *Leadership and Management in Healthcare* and *Practice Teaching in Healthcare* textbooks. I have also had chapters published in edited books and a range of peer-reviewed articles.

# Acknowledgements

I would like to acknowledge the support and constructive comments provided by the commissioning editors at SAGE Publications, and I am also thankful to my daughters Hema, Sheila and Neeta for their support with this venture.

# List of Abbreviations

| | |
|---|---|
| ACE | Accreditation of Clinical Educators |
| AHP | Allied health professions |
| CAIPE | Centre for Advancement of Interprofessional Education |
| CINAHL | Cumulative Index to Nursing and Allied Health Literature |
| CLES+T | Clinical Learning Environment, Supervision and Nurse Teacher |
| CODP | College of Operating Department Practitioners |
| COT | College of Occupational Therapists |
| CPD | Continuing professional development |
| CPT | Community Practice Teachers |
| CQC | Care Quality Commission |
| CSP | Chartered Society of Physiotherapy |
| DDA | Disability Discrimination Act |
| DH | Department of Health |
| EBHC | Evidence-based healthcare |
| EBP | Evidence-based practice |
| ESC | Essential skills clusters |
| GMC | General Medical Council |
| GP | General practitioner |
| HEI | Higher education institute/institution |
| HPC | Health Professions Council |
| IHI | Institute of Healthcare Improvement |
| IPE | Inter-professional education |
| IPL | Inter-professional learning |
| LSQ | Learning Style Questionnaire |
| MMP | Measuring mentorship potential |
| NCIHE | National Committee of Inquiry into Higher Education |
| NHS III | NHS Institute for Innovation and Improvement |
| NHS KSF | NHS Knowledge and Skills Framework |
| NICE | National Institute of Health and Clinical Excellence |
| NMC | Nursing and Midwifery Council |
| NVQ | National Vocational Qualifications |

| | |
|---|---|
| OAR | Ongoing achievement record |
| ODP | Operating department practitioners |
| OPSI | Office of Public Sector Information |
| OSCE | Objective Structured-Simulated Clinical Examination |
| PDP | Personal development plan |
| PDSA | Plan–Do–Study–Act |
| PEF | Practice education facilitators |
| PREP | Post-registration education and practice |
| QAA | Quality Assurance Agency for Higher Education |
| QIPP | Quality, Innovation, Productivity and Prevention |
| RAPSIES | Recognition, Analysis, Preparation, Strategies, Implementation, Evaluation Sustaining (framework) |
| RCN | Royal College of Nursing |
| RCT | Randomised controlled trial |
| RM | Registered midwife |
| RN | Registered nurse |
| SCOPME | Standing Committee on Postgraduate Medical and Dental Education |
| SCPHN | Specialist community public health nurse |
| SEN | Special education need |
| SHA | Strategic Health Authority |
| SMART | Specific, measurable, achievable, realistic and time-limited |
| SOP | Standards of proficiency |
| STEP | Social, technological, economic and political |
| SWOT | Strengths, weaknesses, opportunities and threats |
| UKCC | United Kingdom Central Council for Nursing, Midwifery and Health Visiting |
| VARK | Visual, aural, read–write and kinaesthetic |
| WBL | Work-based learning |

# Introduction

## The Rationale and Scope of this Book

Mentoring has become a significant dimension of professional life in nursing and midwifery (and for some individuals, in their personal lives), particularly in relation to supporting educational preparation of healthcare professionals. Also known by other titles such as 'clinical educator' and 'clinical instructor' in other healthcare professions, and in non-UK countries, formal educational preparation is required in nursing and midwifery to enable mentors to perform this role competently.

Several definitions of this role have evolved over the years, and various research findings on mentoring in different professions published. Mentoring was redefined in a Department of Health (2001a) publication especially as a result of research findings by Philips et al. (2000), extending the role beyond facilitation of practice-based learning during student practice placements to assessment of students' practice competence. The Nursing and Midwifery Council (NMC) (2008a) has retained a very similar definition in its *Standards to Support Learning and Assessment in Practice*, indicating that the mentor is a 'registrant who … facilitates learning, and supervises and assesses students in practice settings' (2008a: 45).

Although the standards for mentors in the NMC (2008a) publication are for registered nurses (RN) and registered midwives (RM) (from here on all healthcare professionals registered with the NMC or the Health Professions Council (HPC) will be referred to as 'registrants'), they are based on general principles of mentoring (or clinical education) so that they are fully applicable to the other three groups of health and social care professions, namely allied health professions (AHP), social work and medicine. In the current scene of inter-professional learning, reciprocal mentoring between health professions has already been happening, where permissible, for at least a decade.

The NMC standards also identify the criteria for becoming a mentor, and the requirements for educational preparation programmes (or courses) for the mentor's role, as well as for the other learning support roles of sign-off mentor, practice teacher and qualified teacher (e.g. nurse lecturer). Furthermore, the standards provide details of the specific competencies (or outcomes) that are required to fulfil the roles of mentor, practice teacher and 'Teacher'. The requirement to maintain a local register of healthcare professionals in these learning support roles and for continuing professional development are also detailed by the NMC.

Mentoring is a widely taught topic, and mentorship courses are provided by most universities offering healthcare courses. Furthermore, for a number of reasons, which include increased appreciation of the value of learning in practice settings for pre-registration nursing students and inter-professional learning, there is an increased demand for mentors, and universities are asked to provide more diverse mentorship education programmes, for example by e-learning. This book explores in detail the standards, competence areas and outcomes for effective mentoring.

To do so, the book draws on contemporary knowledge on the dynamics of mentoring, and research and policies, and aims to enable registrants to acquire the knowledge and skills that are necessary to fulfil all NMC (2008a) standards for mentors. It thus brings together and builds on existing knowledge on principles and practices of mentoring in various arenas, and updates it to current-day mentoring requirements in health and social care. It thus constitutes a firm backdrop for healthcare professionals further to develop and enhance their mentoring expertise.

Recently qualified healthcare professionals who might not yet be functioning in a formal mentoring capacity (associate mentors, for instance) should also find this book useful, as also might more experienced qualified health professionals who either haven't completed a mentoring course, or who were prepared for the role through a previous 'teaching and assessing' course.

This book is a direct result of my numerous years of experience of teaching and examining on mentoring and 'teaching and assessing' courses, as well as a registered nurse in adult nursing and mental health nursing, along with the need for a textbook that reflects current policies and research on mentoring. In addition to current knowledge in the field, this text also recognises the challenges facing both newly qualified and more experienced healthcare professionals whose roles incorporate imparting their clinical knowledge and skills to their juniors and learners quite soon after qualifying, and within resource constraints, role changes and changing healthcare workforce profile. It takes into account day-to-day and longer-term issues and challenges in mentoring, and explores potential solutions, where possible supporting them with relevant theories and current research base. The ensuing implications with regards to responsibility and accountability are also necessarily explored.

# The Structure of this Book

As just indicated, this book is firmly based on current knowledge in the field, and is structured to ensure that it also addresses all NMC's (2008a) standards for mentors. These standards, which can apply to other healthcare professions as well, are based on the recognition that all RNs' and RMs' roles include teaching and supporting learning. Then, approximately a year after qualifying as a healthcare professional, they would participate in an educational preparation programme for the mentor role, some years afterwards for the practice teacher role, and later perhaps for the 'Teacher' role. The NMC refers to this continuum as a developmental framework for supporting learning.

Standards for mentors and other teachers have been available for almost two decades. They have been revised a few times, and the NMC's *Standards to Support Learning and Assessment in Practice* policy document was published in 2006, followed by its second edition in 2008. These now established standards are detailed under eight revised domains of competence and associated different outcomes for mentors, practice teachers and qualified teachers. Universities have been implementing these standards in their mentoring programmes since 2007. This textbook focuses on the content of the eight domain areas identified by the NMC (2008a) and the outcomes for mentors.

*Chapter 1* begins by examining mentoring as a theme in its own right. It starts by identifying the exact nature of the term 'mentor', and differentiates it from other similar or overlapping roles. It thus examines role boundaries between various healthcare learning facilitation roles such as preceptors, clinical supervisors, practice teachers, link tutors and practice education facilitators (PEF), and mentoring in allied health professions. The common aim of all these roles is to facilitate healthcare profession students and learners to develop clinical competence and knowledge during practice placements.

A range of different rationales for the mentoring role are then identified, which is followed by the factors that enable mentors to fulfil this role effectively, including the modes of communication needed for building effective working relationships by mentors, with their learners. Subsequently, the necessary personal and professional attributes of mentors that enable and support the development of learners' clinical skills, including being role models, are explored. The nature and detrimental effects of poor or adverse mentoring are also discussed, followed by an examination of different models of effective mentoring.

Having identified the crucial role that mentoring occupies in enabling learning in practice settings, *Chapter 2* takes a detailed look at how learning occurs. It examines why and what learners learn, significant different perspectives on learning, teaching and education, and learning theories, styles and approaches, as well as the special education needs of students with disabilities.

*Chapter 3* builds on these dimensions of the concept, and explores facilitation of learning. The chapter starts by ascertaining the range of people whom healthcare professionals teach, followed by the reasons for teaching and learning. It then focuses on how healthcare students learn patient or service user care delivery skills in practice settings, and how the mentor utilises opportunities for informal teaching.

The concept facilitation of learning, as distinct from the teaching concept, is examined, followed by key perceptions, and major views, approaches and styles of teaching including andragogy. The levels and stages of skill acquisition (taxonomy levels) are explored, and the types of knowledge associated with skills, e.g. practical knowledge and theoretical knowledge, are considered, along with levels of theory acquisition.

Steps in lesson planning for structured short teaching sessions for teaching skills and knowledge on a one-to-one level, or for teaching small groups of learners or peers, are then discussed. This is followed by an examination of different teaching or presentation methods, and the use of different teaching aids. A discussion follows on some of the more common difficulties that mentors might encounter during short structured teaching sessions, and the likely solutions for them.

Following on from facilitation of learning, *Chapter 4* focuses on the attributes that make practice settings effective learning environments, maintaining which is also a key area of the mentor role (Darling, 1984; NMC, 2008a). The NMC indicates that the mentor should create and develop opportunities for students to identify and undertake experiences to meet their learning needs. Students' perspectives on practice placements such as their own expectations, and their practice objectives are considered followed by an examination of the part played by national guidelines and current policy documents on practice placements. Issues related to practice placements are also examined.

Research related to practice learning environments, which underpins the development of the tool for annual educational audits of practice placement areas, is then examined. Educational audits include ascertaining the psychosocial ethos and the availability of learning resources (human and material) for facilitation of the acquisition of practice competencies by healthcare profession students. The utilisation of learning pathways (based on patient journeys), which can be incorporated in learning contracts, and can play an important role in ensuring the success of the placement is also explored, as well as the concept of work-based learning.

Fundamental to mentorship are evidence-based practice (EBP), research implementation, practice development and management of change. Therefore how the mentor engages with these activities constitutes the focus of *Chapter 5*, as research by Darling (1984) for instance, and also the NMC (2008a) standards for mentorship, firmly indicate that the role of the mentor incorporates full awareness and close monitoring by the mentor of their own standards of patient or service user care.

It is therefore incumbent upon the mentor, especially as role models for mentees, to practise evidence-based care, which they can do by utilising various sources of evidence such as electronic databases where systematically reviewed research evidence is stored. Hierarchies of evidence are therefore examined in detail, along with identifying, critical evaluation, implementation and dissemination of research findings.

One of the principal purposes of mentor education programmes is to equip course participants with the capability to assess students' clinical competence. Ongoing assessment of competence of healthcare practitioners is a fundamental component of the mentor role, and therefore is a component of all educational programmes for skill-based healthcare professions, and this is the area that *Chapter 6* focuses on.

To fulfil this key mentor function effectively, the mentor needs to know and understand the principles and processes of assessment, i.e. what assessments are, the reasons for assessment of competence, who assesses, when and how they are conducted. As to what assessments are, various definitions of assessment are examined, together with the specific aims of assessments. Before assessing the learner's competencies, the mentor needs to plan carefully a placement learning programme for the mentee, and have a good understanding of how to assess and implement approved assessment procedures.

Under how to assess, the chapter explores key principles of assessments, including dimensions of assessment, as well as levels and fairness of assessments. Student self-assessment and peer assessment are also explored. Validity and reliability as crucial attributes of assessments are then explored in some detail, the aim being to ascertain the assessee's fitness to practise. Furthermore, the utilisation of policies and procedures in the management of assessments is explored, along with techniques for giving useful feedback, and documentation of assessments. Pass or fail criteria are examined followed by the signing-off proficiency role.

Recent research findings have highlighted various day-to-day problems encountered by both mentors and students related to assessment of competence during practice placements. Therefore, the mentor needs to exercise leadership, which includes forward planning to avert problems of assessment. *Chapter 7* delves into the details of various potential problems that could occur with assessments, such as those detailed by Phillips et al. (2000) and Gainsbury (2010), and how they should be prevented or resolved. The ethical and legal implications of assessments are also examined.

The mentor's accountability, responsibility and the use of 'professional judgement' are also addressed in the context of the mentor's leadership role. Supporting the student, who is generally perceived as struggling to progress with their placement learning, is also examined, including the role of action plans, and reassessment of the learner. Monitoring ways in which intra- and inter-mentor reliability are achieved, is also explored.

The facilitation of learning and assessment of learners' competence are therefore essential components of the mentor role. *Chapter 8* concentrates on the evaluation of these components. The nature and purpose of evaluation amount to the mentor self-monitoring the quality of their mentoring. The chapter therefore considers what evaluation is, who is involved in evaluation of learning facilitation and assessment, and how it is performed, including the use of models of evaluation. The challenges of facilitation of learning and assessment are examined, followed by an examination of the mentor's ongoing professional development, incorporating details of continuing professional development, mentor updates and triennial reviews and lifelong learning.

Each chapter in the book begins by identifying the chapter content under an introduction that includes chapter outcomes, the main text and a chapter summary. A logical combination of text, illustrations, activities, think points and some case studies are incorporated to engage the reader fully with the material in the book.

## How to Use this Book

This book examines the knowledge base, skills and attitudes required for mentoring, and the NMC's standards for mentors. The text therefore explores theories and research on mentoring, analyses their strengths and weaknesses and examines how they can be applied to day-to-day mentoring and clinical practice activities.

This textbook adopts an analytical and interactive style, with a clear focus on the means of application of theories and principles to various practice settings. Therefore, throughout the book, the reader is encouraged, through activities and think points, to explore and apply concepts to their own practice and roles. The activities usually ask the reader to consider a particular point or component and make some notes, whilst think points ask the reader to reflect on their own experience and knowledge prior to moving on to the next theme in the text. Consequently, the reader needs to interact with the text for optimum benefit. It also allows mentors to exercise freedom and scope to be creative in enabling mentees' learning and assessment of their competence.

The case studies are incorporated as examples of situations that the mentor might encounter, the aim of which is for the reader to explore ways in which they can manage the situation satisfactorily. Furthermore, the information in some of the boxes, for example Box 4.1, is derived from a number of workshops on mentor preparation programmes. As events evolve, and because different practice settings have their own specific requirements and strengths, feel free to make further notes of your own on other components in addition to those in the boxes.

The term 'healthcare professionals' is used in the text to signify all healthcare employees, medical and non-medical, including nurses and allied health professionals who hold a qualification that is recognised by either their national regulatory body or professional body. The term 'registrant' refers to healthcare professionals on either the NMC or HPC professional register. The term 'learner' is used to refer to everyone who wants or needs to learn healthcare skills, whilst 'students' are those learners who are actually following a professional education programme leading to a university qualification.

# 1
# Effective Mentoring

## Introduction

One of the key mechanisms for facilitating learning for healthcare profession students while on practice placements is mentoring. This mechanism is pretty much well established now, and is indeed a very important component of pre-registration education programmes, albeit using a handful of different titles by different health and social care professions. Policy documents such as *Standards to Support Learning and Assessment in Practice* (NMC, 2008a) provide firm indication of the criteria that healthcare professionals have to meet to use the title 'mentor', and details the capabilities that they need to fulfil the role effectively. The first chapter of this book focuses on mentoring as a concept in its own right, defines and differentiates it from similar and overlapping roles and titles, examines the various reasons for mentoring and explores how to mentor effectively. It also examines poor mentoring and how it can be redressed.

## Chapter outcomes

On completion of this chapter, you should be able to:

1  Distinguish between mentoring and similar roles that support learning for healthcare profession students and learners.
2  Explain a range of reasons for requiring mentors for facilitating students' acquisition of professional competence and the associated knowledge base in practice settings.
3  Identify and evaluate a number of factors that can enable effective mentoring, including the characteristics of effective mentors, and the ability to build sound mentor–mentee 'working' relationships.
4  Analyse the likelihood and effects of poor or adverse mentoring, and the actions that can be taken where it is likely to occur.
5  Analyse a number of approaches, guidelines and frameworks for enabling informed and systematic mentoring.

The chapter thus examines a wide range of perspectives on mentoring itself, and also focuses on the NMC's (2008a: 50) domain 'establishing effective working relationships'. The related mentor competence is: 'Demonstrate effective relationship building skills sufficient to support learning, as part of a wider inter-professional team, for a range of students in both practice and academic learning environments'; and the NMC's outcomes for this competence are:

- Demonstrate an understanding of factors that influence how students integrate into practice settings.
- Provide ongoing and constructive support to facilitate transition from one learning environment to another.
- Have effective professional and interprofessional working relationships to support learning for entry to the register.

## The Concept of 'Mentoring'

'Mentoring' as a concept and practice that is related to facilitating professional learning in healthcare has evolved consistently since the 1970s and was formally implemented in pre-registration nursing and midwifery education in the 1980s. Slightly different titles and terminologies are used by different healthcare professional groups for this role, and different definitions have been offered over time as research and expert opinions have influenced the forms in which it is currently utilised.

It is generally well documented, for example in the *Shorter Oxford English Dictionary* (Brown, 2002: 1747), that the term 'mentor' originates from the Greek classical story, *The Odyssey*, in which King Odysseus called upon a trusted friend named Mentor to act as the guide and advisor to his young son Telemachus when he left for another country to fight a war. The word mentor also relates to the Latin word '*mens*' that is, pertaining to, or occurring in the mind (Simpson and Weiner, 1989: 614). The term has gradually evolved to signify a designated person who dedicates some of their time to help individuals to learn during their developmental years, to progress towards and achieve maturity and establish their identity. It has been implemented as a formal role in nurse education to direct focus on enabling students to gain safe and effective clinical practice skills during practice placements. This section disentangles the concept of mentor from similar titles by exploring the differences and similarities between them.

### Distinguishing between the mentor's and related roles

The mentor role is just one of several that support learning in practice settings, and therefore there is some overlap in certain aspects of such roles, such as in the characteristics of the appropriate personnel who support learning, but there are distinct boundaries as well. A study conducted by Carnwell et al. (2007), for instance, to explore the likely differences in the roles of mentors, lecturer-practitioners and link tutors indicate that mentors tend to focus principally on individual students, lecturer-practitioners on the 'learning environment', and link tutors on knowledge acquisition and fulfilling course requirements.

---

### Activity 1.1   Different education support roles and functions

To begin with, make notes on what you think are the meanings and functions of the following roles: mentor, preceptor, clinical supervisor, assessor and other similar roles you have encountered, and the differences between them.

---

You are likely to have identified a variety of roles that enable or support learning for students and other learners in practice settings, which might include practice facilitators and even the university-based course tutor. Thus, although there are common elements in the definitions, scope and remit of mentor and similar roles, there are also differences. The most popular learning support roles are examined next.

### Mentor

Beside the helping function during developmental years indicated by dictionary definitions of the term *mentor,* as a result of research by Phillips et al. (2000) on behalf of the then English National Board for Nursing, Midwifery and Health Visiting, the Department of Health (DH) (2001a: 6) redefined the mentor as 'a nurse, midwife or health visitor who facilitates learning, super-vises and assesses students in the clinical setting'. Prior to this, the mentor was a registrant who facilitated learning, and the assessor was another registrant who assessed students' competencies.

Mentor is defined similarly by the NMC (2008a: 45) as a registrant who has met the outcomes of Stage 2 (i.e. those of a qualified mentor) and who facilitates learning, and supervises and assesses students in practice settings. The DH's (2001a) definition resulted from a range of issues related to men-toring and assessing pre-registration student nurses and midwives during practice placements that had been identified by Phillips et al.'s (2000) research and other earlier studies (e.g. White et al., 1993). At that time, Spouse (2001a) found that the terms 'mentorship', 'preceptorship' and 'supervision' were being used synonymously, while White et al. (1993) had earlier found that mentors themselves were unclear about their roles due to insufficient educational preparation.

Going beyond definitions of mentor, the NMC (2008a) identifies a range of day-to-day functions of the mentor in terms of 26 outcomes that are grouped under eight domains (which form the major focus of this book). However, research on mentoring (e.g. by Kerry and Mayes, 1995) indicate that definitions of mentor need to include:

- nurturing;
- role modelling;
- functioning (as teacher, sponsor, encourager, counsellor and friend);
- focusing on the professional development of the mentee; and
- sustaining a caring relationship over time.

A concept analysis of the mentor role by Billay and Yonge (2004: 573) across several health, non-health and social care professions indicates that its defining attributes include 'being a role model, being a facilitator, having good communication skills, being knowledgeable about the field of expertise, and needing to understand the principles of adult education'.

It has to be noted at this point that although the term mentor is clearly defined in UK policy documents, in particular by the NMC (2008a) and the DH (2001a), mentor is defined differently in nursing in other countries, such as in Canada (Billay and Yonge, 2004), and even in the UK in the medical profession (General Medical Council (GMC), 2010), in that it refers to qualified healthcare professionals being mentored by more experienced mutually selected colleagues. Also, in some UK professions, e.g. psychologists, the term 'protégé' is used when referring to the mentee (e.g. Barnett, 2008).

## Preceptor

As the term most closely related to mentor, the NMC (2006a) identifies *preceptors* as first-level registrants who have had at least 12 months' (or equivalent) experience within the same area of practice as the practitioner requiring support, and will normally have completed a mentor or practice teacher educational preparation programme. The NMC indicates that the preceptor and the preceptee should agree between themselves the nature of their working relationship and the desired outcomes. It should be noted, however, that preceptorship is not clinical supervision, which in the UK refers to structured peer support for, and by, registrants throughout their careers.

The preceptor role emerged from the realisation that for newly qualified nurses, the transition from being a student to becoming a registered healthcare professional is a major leap in responsibility and accountability. It is partly based on an earlier study by Kramer (1974) who found that the first few months after qualifying were often marked by dramatically conflicting value systems, between the aims of pre-registration education and the reality of day-to-day nursing. This led to high attrition rates among newly qualified nurses. Various studies reveal such concerns even today.

The NMC (2006a) recommends preceptorship for all newly qualified registrants, for RNs changing their area of practice and for qualified nurses from other European Economic Area states and other countries. It indicates that for preceptorship to be effective, it should last approximately four months, and recommends that the preceptor should:

- Facilitate the transition of the 'new registrant' from student to a registrant who is confident, effective and up to date with their practice and knowledge.
- Provide feedback to the preceptee on those nursing or midwifery interventions that they are performing safely and effectively, and those that they aren't (if any).
- Facilitate the preceptee to achieve the standards, competencies or objectives set by the employer for new registrants.

Structured preceptorship programmes are devised locally by trusts or their departments and are normally of four to six months' duration, and often include the specialism-specific competencies in the induction programmes for the particular practice setting, which, when achieved, the preceptee can incorporate into their professional portfolio.

More recently, wide availability of preceptorship has been gaining momentum since publication of the Darzi Report (DH, 2008a), and healthcare trusts have since created new roles such as Preceptorship Co-ordinator to establish this mechanism. Dedicated government funding is now available on a recurring basis to provide preceptorship to all newly qualified nurses (e.g. Bayley and Bayliss-Pratt, 2010). Neither the Darzi Report nor the NMC (2006a) identify the specific content of preceptorship programmes, which are therefore adaptable according to local needs.

However, drawing partly on the successful implementation of preceptorship in Scotland through the *Flying Start* (Scottish Government, 2010) pilot schemes, which started in 2006, the DH (2010a: 11) redefines preceptorship as: 'A period of structured transition for the newly registered practitioner during which he or she will be supported by a preceptor, to develop their confidence as an autonomous professional, refine skills, values and behaviours and to continue on their journey of lifelong learning.' It identifies a preceptor as: 'a registered practitioner who has been given a formal responsibility to support a newly registered practitioner through preceptorship' (2010a: 6). The DH presents a framework for effective preceptoring, within which it also identifies the 'attributes' of an effective preceptor – see Box 1.1.

## Box 1.1   Attributes of the effective preceptor

- Gives constructive feedback
- Sets goals and assesses competency
- Facilitates problem-solving
- Utilises active listening skills
- Shows understanding and ably engages in reflective practice in the working environment
- Demonstrates good time-management and leadership skills
- Prioritises care
- Demonstrates appropriate clinical decision-making and evidence-based practice
- Recognises their own limitations and those of others
- Knows what resources are available and how to refer a newly registered practitioner appropriately if additional support is required
- Is an effective and inspirational role model and demonstrates professional values, attitude and behaviours
- Demonstrates a clear understanding of the regulatory impact of the care that they deliver and the ability to pass on this knowledge
- Provides a high standard of practice at all times

*Source*: DH (2010a)

The College of Occupational Therapists (COT) (2009: 8–9) suggests four preceptorship standards that should be addressed in these programmes, namely working with clients, working with colleagues, written communication and health and safety policies. Professional development needs to be achieved in conjunction with *NHS Knowledge and Skills Framework* (*NHS KSF*) (DH, 2004a) dimensions along with indicators that progress through the four levels that can then form the basis for developmental activities for individual occupational therapists, which is also congruous with competencies that they will require for their future careers.

Furthermore, the NMC (2009a) is exploring the appropriateness and feasibility of whether the point of completion of the preceptorship programme can comprise the point of 'validation' for the healthcare professional when they have their name and qualification entered on the NMC's register, which can subsequently be followed up by regular re-validation at re-registration points.

### Assessor
The term 'assessor' remains in use and is often used to denote a role similar to that of the mentor but solely with the assessment component (DH, 2001a).

It usually refers to an appropriately qualified and experienced healthcare professional who has undertaken relevant educational preparation to develop skills in assessing students' level of attainment related to the stated practice competencies (e.g. National Vocational Qualifications (NVQ) assessor).

## Clinical educator

The role of the clinical educator is akin to mentoring and is generally used by some healthcare professions such as medicine and physiotherapy for facilitating student learning during practice placements. In physiotherapy, for instance, a clinical educator is 'A qualified practitioner who directly supports a student's learning during clinical education/practice-based learning. It also applies to the clinician's education role in relation to other learners (for example junior staff)' (Chartered Society of Physiotherapy (CSP), 2004: 20).

## Clinical supervision

Clinical supervision refers to a peer-support role based on a clinically focused professional relationship between healthcare professionals in which one party is the clinical supervisor and the other the supervisee. The clinical supervisor undergoes educational preparation for this role and utilises clinical knowledge and experience to assist peers to further develop their own knowledge, competence, values and practices.

Waskett (2010: 12) notes that 'many nurses do not have regular, protected access to confidential conversations about the everyday challenges of their work', and amongst the various models of clinical supervision that are available for a systematic approach to this activity is Waskett's 4S model, comprising structure, skills, support and sustainability.

## Clinical supervisor

Clinical supervisor a term used in the context of clinical supervision signifying the provider of peer support to the clinical supervisee. It may be used to identify mentoring-type roles in some healthcare professions or vocations.

## Practice teacher

The title or role of practice teacher was initially specifically adopted in recognition of the additional preparation required for mentoring students on specialist community public health nurses (SCPHN) courses. A practice teacher is therefore 'A registrant who has gained knowledge, skills and competence in both their specialist area of practice and in their teaching role, meeting the outcomes of stage 3, and who facilitates learning, supervises and assesses students in a practice setting' (NMC, 2008a: 46). It refers to specialist areas of practice where they support students undertaking a specialist qualification or at a level beyond initial registration.

Practice teachers therefore facilitate learning and assess post-qualifying students on their achievement of specialism-specific specialist or advanced practice competencies. However, practice teaching, practice learning and student supervision are terms that are also used for mentoring student social workers during practice placements for instance (Shardlow and Doel, 1996).

### Registrant

Both NMC and HPC refer to healthcare professionals who are currently on their respective registers as 'registrants'. Nurse and midwife registrants already have a teaching role towards others in the practice setting by virtue of the competencies that they have achieved as part of pre-registration education programmes, as well as through NMC's (2008b) code of practice, as other healthcare professionals usually do as well.

### Supervision

In this book, the term 'supervision' is used in accordance with its dictionary meaning, which is to direct or oversee the performance, action or work of another, which in this instance refers to the mentor directing and overseeing the mentee's learning. The term does, however, have very specific meaning in the field of counselling, in which it refers to counselling situations wherein one or more highly experienced counsellor helps a less experienced or more junior counsellor develop their practice.

Hawkins and Shohet (2006) refer to supervision as interpersonal inter-action between the identified supervisor and the supervisee, wherein the general goal is to enable the supervisee to become more effective in help-ing people. The British Association for Counselling and Psychotherapy (2010) indicates that all counsellors, psychotherapists, supervisors and their trainers have an obligation to use regular and ongoing supervision to enhance the quality of the services provided and to commit to updating practice by seeking training and other opportunities for continuing profes-sional development, which is also accessed independently of any managerial relationships.

### Supervisor

The term 'supervisor' tends to be used in the context of management of workers to ensure designated tasks are completed, and to a specified stand-ard, rather than in relation to the facilitation of learning. It refers to indi-viduals in the organisation who have authority in the interest of the employer to recruit staff for specified posts, assign duties, oversee the qual-ity of their work and take relevant professional development or disciplinary actions as appropriate.

# Roles of practice education facilitators, personal tutors and link tutors

In addition to the above roles for supporting learning, other roles such as buddy and coach are also emerging (the latter is discussed later in this chapter). More firmed-up roles such as those of facilitators of learning who are fully or partly employed by universities include practice education facilitator (PEF), personal tutor and link tutor.

## Practice education facilitator and practice educator

The PEF role in nursing and midwifery also emerged largely from the study of mentors by Phillips et al. (2000). It is defined by the DH (2001a: 6) as a 'role of the teacher of nursing, midwifery or health visiting who makes a significant contribution to education in the practice setting, co-ordinating student experiences and assessment of learning'. The PEF thus leads the development of practice and provides support and guidance to mentors and others who contribute to the student's learning in practice settings, and achievement of practice competencies.

The educational preparation for the PEF role is usually at postgraduate level. The post is generally funded directly by Strategic Health Authorities (SHA) (SHAs will cease to exist from 2012, and part of their functions will be taken over by the NHS Commissioning Board (DH, 2010b)) and generally entails practice-based teaching four days a week and university-based work one day a week. This is a very important role as PEFs are also called upon to attend to students during practice placements when busy clinical staff are unable to dedicate sufficient extra attention to students who are struggling or failing to progress with their practice placement competencies. For students on practice placements, PEFs might also organise dedicated group discussion sessions away from the practice setting for particular categories of students for reflection and peer support purposes.

There are small differences in the way that the role and title are implemented in different healthcare professions. The College of Radiographers (2006: 7), for instance, adopts the Higher Education Academy (2005: 6) definition of practice educator, which is: 'the identified practitioner in practice placement who facilitates student learning face to face on a daily basis and generally has responsibility for the formative and/or summative assessment of competence'. Thus, the practice educator role in radiography and other AHPs is largely similar to the mentor role in nursing and midwifery, and educational preparation for the practice educator role can take either the experiential learning route or a taught programme of six days' workshops spread over several months (e.g. COT, 2006). In physiotherapy it is a more generic term referring to physiotherapists who teach in practice settings.

As for the PEF role in nursing, in a workshop conducted by the NMC (2009b) on the role of PEFs in the context of the review of pre-registration nursing education, several key priorities were identified, including due regard, accountability and essential skills clusters, and a number of issues as well. However, McArthur and Burns (2008), amongst others, have evaluated the role of PEFs and found that whilst various staff think that PEFs should work with students, the PEFs themselves feel that their main role is in supporting mentors.

Nonetheless, a study by Carlisle et al. (2009: 715) on the impact of the PEF role in Scotland revealed that the PEF role is 'accepted widely across Scotland and is seen as valuable to the development of quality clinical learning environments, providing support and guidance for mentors when dealing with "failing" students, and encouraging the identification of innovative learning opportunities'.

### Personal tutor

Each pre-registration student is allocated to a nurse lecturer who acts as a personal tutor to the student. This role normally lasts for the duration of the three-year pre-registration course and involves:

- Supporting, advising and monitoring students' progress throughout the educational programme.
- Accessing students' practice records for required information, within an ethos of confidentiality and professional accountability.
- Liaising with the mentor, link tutor and student and, where concern is expressed, considering evidence and developing an action plan with the student.

### Link tutor

The link tutor is usually a university lecturer whose responsibility is to assist clinicians in named practice settings. They assist mentors to interpret students' practice competencies and are available to support mentors when required. They might also assist in the development of the practice setting as a more effective learning environment for all learners. Students tend to receive a visit by the link tutor early in the placement, especially first-year students, to ascertain which learning objectives are realistically achievable. Further visits are arranged as required.

Some of the functions of the personal tutor and the link tutor have increasingly become part of the PEF's remit but they continue to provide an essential complementary function.

## Mentoring activities in allied health and social care professions

The role of practice educator in AHPs was examined briefly in the above paragraphs. Naturally enabling students and learners to acquire skills for safe and effective practice prevail in all health and social care professions. In addition to knowledge gained from research and the planned activities of professionals to enable learning, professional and regulatory bodies provide informed guidance on how this can be achieved. The HPC (2008) *Standards of Proficiency – Operating Department Practitioners*, for instance, details the competencies that operating department practitioner (ODP) students have to be competent in to register with the HPC as an ODP.

Furthermore, several healthcare profession organisations publish separate profession specific standards for mentors, such as the College of Operating Department Practitioners' (CODP) (2009) *Standards, Recommendations and Guidance for Mentors and Practice Placements*.

The HPC's (2009) *Standards of Education and Training Guidance* provides guidance on the design of pre-qualifying AHP education curricula, which is supported by specific standards of proficiency (SOP) for each of the 15 allied healthcare professions (e.g. HPC (2008) noted above), that it currently regulates, namely (HPC, 2010):

1   Arts therapists
2   Biomedical scientists
3   Chiropodists/Podiatrists
4   Clinical scientists
5   Dietitians
6   Hearing-aid dispensers
7   Occupational therapists
8   Operating department practitioners
9   Orthoptists
10  Paramedics
11  Physiotherapists
12  Practitioner psychologists
13  Prosthetists/Orthotists
14  Radiographers
15  Speech and language therapists

In addition to the role of the radiography healthcare profession which was referred to earlier in this chapter, the HPC identifies the 'practice placement educator' as 'A person who is responsible for a student's education during their period of clinical or practical experience' (HPC, 2009: 61). It indicates under the standard 'Practice placement educators must have relevant knowledge, skills and experience,' that they should have the knowledge, skills and experience to support students, and provide a safe environment for effective learning. The HPC, however, does not currently set specific requirements about the qualifications and experience that practice placement educators must have to fulfil the role effectively.

Mentoring in physiotherapy has been formalised as clinical educators through the Accreditation of Clinical Educators (ACE) Scheme (CSP, 2004). An evaluation of the ACE Scheme (CSP, 2007) after several hundred physiotherapists had been accredited, suggests that it gives greater recognition to the senior clinicians responsible for student placements; participants believed that they were more reflective and that accredited status had a positive impact on their students, colleagues and patients; and that student placements were planned with more confidence and that staff development was more structured. Formal education preparation for such mentor equivalent roles for all health and social care professions seems imminent.

The titles 'practice placement educator' and 'practice placement co-ordinator' are also utilised in various AHP documents with reference to designated healthcare professionals who provide support and information to clinical educators (akin to the mentor role in nursing and midwifery), and also monitors the standards of practice placement being experienced by students (HPC, 2009).

Hinton (2009) reports on her experiences of mentoring ODP students in which she indicates that it is an activity that is beneficial for students as well as for ODP mentors. On the other hand, Mallik and McGowan (2007) completed a scoping exercise on the nature of practice education in five healthcare professions, namely dietetics, nursing, occupational therapy, physiotherapy and radiography, and concluded that although there are areas of good practice, 'these do so against the provision of well-supported, clearly supervised and adequately quality-assured practice education' (2007: 58). They recommend that such issues should be resolved by the various healthcare professions, and need to be recognised and rewarded, and that collaborative work across the professions should be enhanced for achievement of more well-rounded practice education.

Furthermore, Lloyd-Jones et al. (2007) report on the successful implementation of inter-professional learning (IPL) across the whole curriculum of healthcare profession courses, on campus and in practice settings, and also that it figures in assessment strategies.

On the other hand, Lakasing and Francis (2005) argue that because many nurse lecturers are not active clinicians, this tends to create a theory–practice gap that mentors have to redress during student practice placements, unlike medical academics who are also practising doctors. They indicate that mentors should therefore be provided with protected time and extra remuneration to enable them to fulfil this demanding role more effectively. Where extra funding is made available for mentoring activities, the money can be utilised to employ additional pro rata staff to allow the mentor protected time for more effective mentoring.

Lack of funding for mentorship in general medicine in the USA was also identified in a study by Luckhaupt et al. (2005). However, Barton (2006) reports on a study that explored the experiences of doctors mentoring students on nurse practitioner courses, and concludes that medical mentors (clinical educators) experience conflict in that as the students acquire new clinical skills and roles, this also amounts to the mentors feeling that their traditional medical authority is being challenged. This led to renegotiation of professional boundaries between nurse practitioners and doctors.

In summarising this section on mentor and similar roles, it is clear that there are areas within these roles that overlap, and there are distinctions between them when current national policy and professional bodies' definitions are considered. On the other hand, as these roles evolve and different models of implementation are applied in different settings, endeavouring to disentangle the educational philosophy underlying these roles, such as differentiating between coaching and mentoring, is seen as a 'sterile debate' by Megginson et al. (2006: 5).

## Why do Learners Need Mentors?

The mentor role is widely implemented and utilised and it may now appear to be an obvious facility afforded to learners. A more detailed examination of why we need mentors for mentoring students and learners reveals a number of reasons.

### Activity 1.2   Why mentors?

The idea of this activity is to explore the variety of reasons why mentors are required in healthcare professional education, particularly in the context of the prevailing definition of the term. Therefore, consider and make notes on the question, 'Why do we need mentors (and preceptors) in: (a) nursing, midwifery and allied health professions; and (b) personal life. List as many reasons as you can think of.

When students on mentoring courses are asked to cite as many reasons as they can think of for requiring mentors, they tend to be able to identify several. The reasons given include the need to ensure safe practice by learners, to enable students to achieve their course practice competencies, and to listen and act as a sounding board for any worries or fears or the mentee's ideas on care delivery. Further reasons cited by students for mentoring learners in (a) nursing, midwifery, and allied health professions, and (b) personal life are listed in Box 1.2.

## Box 1.2 Why we need mentors

(a) In nursing and other health professions

- For guidance and support
- To structure working environment for learning
- For constructive and honest feedback
- For debriefing related to good/bad experience during placement
- As a link person with other areas
- As a role model
- To assess competence
- As a friend and counsellor
- For encouragement
- To provide the appropriate knowledge base for nursing interventions
- For questioning
- For protection from poor practice
- To build confidence
- For sharing learning, i.e. learning from each other
- Is an NMC requirement
- To keep own skills and knowledge up to date
- For linking theory to practice
- For developing one's work skills in teaching and explaining
- To provide structured learning programmes during practice placements

(b) In personal life

- For the development of one's self
- To share experiences
- For encouragement
- To build up confidence
- For honest opinions and views
- As a role model (may be a parent figure, etc.)
- For socialisation
- For support and guidance

Another advantage of mentoring is that students who have been on placement in the particular practice setting might apply for a post in that setting after qualifying, i.e. they can have recruitment benefits. Furthermore, van Eps et al. (2006) explored the benefits of mentoring in a study that evaluated students' perceptions of mentorship, and concluded that mentorship does enable the development of competent practice, especially if it is founded on supportive longer-term mentor–mentee relationships.

It could be argued that everyone could benefit from having a 'mentor' in their personal lives, at times referred to as a 'soulmate'. This privileged role is self-selected by both parties and could be fulfilled by a friend, partner, parent or senior peer. It is consistent with the current medical mentoring definition of mentor, which suggests that the mentor is selected by the learner for support and guidance. However, student mentors identify various reasons for the mentoring role. There are also various research and policy reasons for the requirement for this role. The most significant ones for healthcare are now discussed.

Firstly, mentoring has become an increasingly popular concept in a wide range of settings, for example:

- In schools and other educational institutions – for initial teacher training.
- In business – to support personal development of business skills, human resource strategies, and business development and self-employment. Further guidance on business mentoring in the United Kingdom is available from the Institute of Directors.
- In support of young people who are, or are at risk of becoming, disaffected or excluded from society – to raise achievement, self-confidence, personal and social skills.
- Medical mentoring – as for a doctor or medical student receiving guidance from an identified more senior or experienced colleague on a range of work-related matters.
- Management mentoring – incorporates coaching, and is discussed later in this chapter.

Thus, mentoring has already been implemented quite effectively in non-healthcare professions and social contexts. For instance, mentoring has worked successfully in initial teacher training (e.g. Furlong and Maynard, 1995; Kerry and Mayes, 1995) for some time. The concept has developed continuously in this context since then, and international journals such as *Mentoring & Tutoring: Partnership in Learning* report on the latest developments and research on various aspects of the concept. Harrison et al. (2006), for instance, conducted an analysis of mentoring new teachers in secondary schools, and found that 'best practice for "developmental mentoring" involves elements of challenge and risk-taking within supportive school environments with clear induction systems in place and strong school ethos in relation to professional development' (2006: 1055).

Furthermore, Barnett (2008: 3) notes that mentoring new teachers results in benefits for the mentor as well in terms of professional stimulation and collaboration, personal fulfilment, friendship and support, motivation to remain current in one's field and networking opportunities; and benefits to the institution include more satisfied staff and greater scholarly productivity.

As for medical mentoring, whilst in other countries, e.g. the USA, medical mentoring refers to mentoring medical students, in the UK the mentoring relationship is confidential between two doctors, the mentor and the mentee (GMC, 2010: 4; Viney and McKimm, 2010: 107), and is more akin to clinical supervision in nursing, midwifery and AHPs, which was explained earlier in this chapter. For this, doctors adopt the Standing Committee on Postgraduate Medical and Dental Education's (SCOPME) definition of mentoring, which is:

> the process whereby an experienced, highly regarded, empathic individual (the mentor), by listening and talking in confidence, guides another individual, often but not always working in the same organisation or field (the mentee), in the development and re-examination of the mentee's own ideas, learning, personal and professional development. (McKimm et al., 2007: 15)

A second reason for the need for mentoring is that which was identified when nurse education moved into the higher education sector *en masse* during the 1980s and 1990s with the restructured Project 2000 pre-registration curricula and a change in emphasis in certain aspects, and the findings of various research studies on these novel programmes were captured eventually in the UKCC's (1999) *Fitness for Practice* publication. This publication documented the strengths of these programmes, but one of the prominent findings of these studies was that at the point of registration students were not clinically as skilled as those who emerged from pre-Project 2000 programmes. This rein-forced the need for wider availability of competent clinically based mentors to enable students to learn clinical skills so that they are 'fit for practice'.

The *Dearing Report* on learning in higher education, and other related national reports, also strongly advocates that higher education courses should enable students to become fit for practice, fit for purpose and fit for award (National Committee of Inquiry into Higher Education (NCIHE), 1997).

Thirdly, the findings of Kramer's (1974) study mentioned earlier indicated the need for preceptors for newly qualified nurses. The notion was extrapo-lated to pre-registration students and is also a reason for the introduction of the term 'mentor' in the UK in the 1980s as a means of supporting student nurses with their learning during practice placements.

Fourthly, the standards or codes of professional (or good) practice for nurses, doctors, social workers and AHPs usually indicate that qualified practitioners have a duty to 'facilitate students and others to develop their competence' (e.g. NMC, 2008b: 5). Similar requirements feature in healthcare professionals' job descriptions, which are also guided by the *NHS KSF* (DH, 2004a).

Mentoring of course also provides registrants with an opportunity to teach, which in itself is a feature of their own professional development and can constitute a stepping stone in their own career trajectories.

Yet another reason for mentoring is the concept of work-based learning, which constitutes practice-based development of skills and (practical) knowl-edge. Its main features are reflected in the social learning theory which was constituted by Bandura (1986, 1997), and which centres on learning skills by

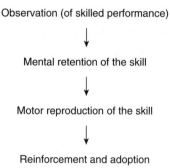

**FIGURE 1.1** The four processes of learning

observing skilled professionals perform them first. Social learning theory therefore also involves mentors being role models, and comprises four processes of learning (see Figure 1.1).

In more detail, the four processes of learning that the learner goes through are:

1   *Observation of skilled performance*

Individual observes a skilled performance ('modelling stimulus').
The observed behaviour is seen as useful and distinctive.
Observer's level of arousal pertaining to the skill is raised.
Observer is keen to learn the skill.
Observer has previously felt positive reinforcement for learning skills.

2   *Mental retention of the skill*

Step-by-step performance of the skill is mentally assimilated.
Mental rehearsal of modelled behaviour.

3   *Motor reproduction of the skill*

Observer carries out observed behaviour or skill, and self-evaluates it in terms of performance.

4   *Reinforcement and adoption*

The behaviour is reinforced by external reward such as praise or through self-reinforcement, and is likely to be adopted.

According to Bandura (1986), we do not possess any inherent behaviour patterns at birth except reflexes, and therefore learning occurs by observing other people, which is the essence of social learning theory, and which therefore includes learning from social situations. In healthcare, learners (mentees and preceptees) learn and acquire practical skills from mentors and other healthcare professionals through the four processes identified in Figure 1.1.

Bandura's (1986) social learning theory had previously been termed 'observational learning' or 'modelling', and was built on behaviourist learning theory (see Chapter 2). It is a component of work-based learning, a concept that is examined in detail in Chapter 4 in the context of learning in practice settings.

Yet another reason for mentoring is that it can be effective in management mentoring, which is an activity wherein trainee managers are mentored by named highly experienced managers to enable those less experienced to develop their management skills (e.g. Megginson et al., 2006). Waters et al. (2003), for instance, report on a very successful tailored mentoring programme for newly appointed nurse managers where mentees can choose their mentors.

---

### Activity 1.3   Management mentoring

All nurses and the majority of healthcare professionals have a management and organisation of care role. Some healthcare professionals opt to develop their careers as clinical managers. Explore with a band 6 colleague how management mentoring is utilised informally, and possibly formally, to enable healthcare professionals to develop as clinical managers.

---

Brooke and Ham (2003) also report on a successful programme that enables managers to develop their leadership skills. A small number of healthcare professionals have had experience of management mentoring, which on occasion is referred to as management coaching. This is a longer-term role than mentoring pre-registration students on practice placement. The management mentor role can initially take the form of a coach that advises the mentee to explore utilisation of particular management techniques, and takes a more directive approach. When the mentee has developed substantial management skills, the role can become more akin to a mentor's, i.e. less directive; and much later mentor–mentee activities become more akin to those of 'buddies', i.e. equals.

## Mentoring and coaching

Other learning support roles that utilise aspects of the mentor's have been identified by various agents, some of which are still developing, and include *practice facilitator, buddy, coach* and *co-tutor*. The term 'coach' tends to surface sporadically in nursing. This, however, is a term and title that is more closely linked to sports, which involves training individuals to enhance their physical performance so that they are able to take part in competitions in specific sports; and in the context of life coaching. In both instances, coaching implies one-to-one guidance and support for enhancement of one or more specific skills, as also identified by Coleman and Glover (2010) in the context of leadership skills. Nonetheless, it is also increasingly associated with more experienced healthcare managers and executives enabling more junior staff (at times referred to as pupils) to develop skills that can enhance their management and leadership performance in the organisation. The GROW (also referred to as GROWing – which stands for Goal, Reality, Options, Will/Wrap up) model is advocated (e.g. Connor and Pokora, 2007) as a framework for effective coaching.

## Who can be a Mentor?

Despite all the reasons for mentoring discussed so far, it shouldn't be taken for granted that all qualified healthcare professionals wish to undertake mentoring work, for all or even some of the time. Some healthcare professionals feel that continuous allocation of students to them all year round can be detrimental to their own effectiveness with their workloads, and they would like some space for reflection and to focus on their own professional development.

In the selection of mentors, it is important to ensure that they have the necessary skills and expertise for mentoring, which according to Neary (2000a) include coaching, counselling, facilitating, setting standards, assessing and giving feedback. Other writers and researchers identify similar lists of skills. Such lists initially appear simplistic as a whole range of expertise is required to undertake the mentorship role, and this can usually be developed through appropriate educational preparation.

In some professions, such as in medicine in the UK, the very definition of mentor suggests that students should be able to select their mentor. However, in reality, in healthcare professions, students on practice placement do not usually have the opportunity to select their mentors due to various factors such as RNs' increased workload. Nonetheless, there are situations when mentees are encouraged to or have the option to choose their mentor, such as if they go back to a particular practice setting for a second placement later in their course.

There are occasions when RNs may be able to select one individual to whom they can relate throughout an entire programme as a personal mentor or a 'buddy'. On the other hand, the NMC (2008a) also identifies the criteria for who can be mentors for nursing and midwifery students, which are as follows:

• Be registered in the same part or sub-part of the register as the student they are to assess and, for the nurses' part of the register, be in the same field of practice (adult, mental health, learning disability or children's nursing).

- Have developed their own knowledge, skills and competence beyond registration, and have been registered for at least one year.
- Have successfully completed an NMC-approved mentor preparation programme, or a similar previous programme.
- Have the ability to select, support and assess a range of learning opportunities in their area of practice for students undertaking NMC-approved programmes.
- Be able to support learning in an inter-professional environment – selecting and supporting a range of learning opportunities for students from other professions.
- Have the ability to contribute to the assessment of other professionals under the supervision of an experienced assessor from that profession.
- Be able to make judgements about [the] competence of NMC students on the same part of the register, and in the same field of practice, and be accountable for such decisions.
- Be able to support other nurses and midwives in meeting CPD needs in accordance with *The Code: Standards of Conduct, Performance and Ethics for Nurses and Midwives* (NMC, 2008b).

These criteria clearly imply that not all registrants are suitable for mentoring, at least not for all categories of learners. The competencies and outcomes for mentors are discussed next.

## How to Mentor

The principles and methods of mentoring incorporate a number of factors that are essential for effective student learning. They include meeting NMC's (2008a) standards for mentors that are identified under eight domains, these being:

1   Establishing effective working relationships.
2   Facilitation of learning.
3   Assessment and accountability.
4   Evaluation of learning.
5   Creating an environment for learning.
6   Context of practice.
7   Evidence-based practice.
8   Leadership.

The first domain, 'establishing effective working relationships', encompasses:

- How effective working relationships are developed and maintained.
- Effective mentor–mentee communication.
- Characteristics of the mentor.
- Actions by the mentor that support learning, including the use of learning contracts.

Each of the other domains is addressed separately in subsequent chapters as detailed in the introduction to this book.

## Effective working relationships

In a study conducted by Johansson et al. (2010) to measure the quality of teaching and learning in practice settings using a scale known as CLES+T (Clinical Learning Environment, Supervision and Nurse Teacher), it emerged that the supervisory relationship (8 items on the scale out of 34) between mentor and mentee is the most important factor contributing to clinical learning experiences. However, for two individuals who are usually initially unknown to each other, adopting the mentor–mentee roles presupposes that they are able to communicate with each other, develop a rapport and cultivate a 'working' relationship at the very least. The word *rapport* means 'a state of deep spiritual, emotional or mental connection between people', including understanding and empathy (Brown, 2002: 2465), and *relationship* refers to 'the state or fact of being related, an emotional association between two people' (Brown, 2002: 2520).

The requirement for effective working relationships is recognised by the NMC (2008a). But how are relationships formed between two designated parties? According to Rogers and Freiberg (1994), counsellors and helpers build a trusting and working relationship by ensuring first of all that certain key conditions prevail. These conditions are:

- Acceptance (or unconditional positive regard) – of the individual for who they are, that is, for their individual strengths and weaknesses; and mutual respect.
- Genuineness – as a person, honesty.
- Empathic understanding – being able and willing to view situations from the other person's perspective.

These key conditions are explored in some detail in the context of student-centred learning in Chapter 3. Rogers and Freiberg (1994) emphasise that 'trust' underpins these key conditions, which they suggest in reality permeate all mutually beneficial relationships. It is akin to a 'psychological contract' between the mentor and mentee, or between patient and carer, or colleagues and friends. The two parties also have to be willing to spend time together to maintain this relationship, and to work towards the achievement of practice objectives, for instance. Although the mentee has actively to seek out relevant learning opportunities, the mentor also needs to take actions that support the mentee's learning, for example by familiarising themselves adequately with the mentee's educational programme.

## Effective mentor–mentee communication

The skills and techniques of communication are some of the most important tools the practitioner undertaking the mentoring role has to utilise. The healthcare professional is normally already a skilled communicator in healthcare settings through initial educational preparation, and therefore it is important to establish which other communication techniques they need to develop to extend their skillbase. Effective communication skills are essential within all teaching and learning situations. So what is communication?

The word 'communication' originates from the Latin word *communicare* which means to impart, share, convey or exchange information (Brown, 2002: 463). It is 'a complex, ongoing dynamic process in which the participants simultaneously create shared meaning in an interaction. The goal of communication is to approach, as closely as possible, a common understanding of the message sent, and the one received' (Sullivan and Decker, 2009: 122). Furthermore, the factors influencing communication are:

- Past conditioning.
- The present situation.
- Each person's purpose in the communication.
- Each person's attitudes towards self, the topic, and each other.

Various modes of communication are available to the mentor to choose from, including:

- Written, for example handwritten, typed, emailed, faxed, printed.
- Oral (spoken), for example face to face, one to one, in groups, by telephone.
- Non-verbal, for example body posture, eye contact, tone of voice.

Oral (spoken) communication is always accompanied by non-verbal messages, vocal and non-vocal. In fact, non-verbal hues are more powerful than verbal messages. Furthermore, Argyle (1994) suggests that non-verbal signals of a friendly attitude (as opposed to an unfriendly attitude) are:

- *Proximity*: closer, leaning forward if seated.
- *Orientation*: more direct, but side to side for some situations.
- *Gaze*: more gaze for each other, and mutual gaze.
- *Facial expression*: more smiling.
- *Gestures*: head nods, lively movements.
- *Posture*: open arms stretched towards each other rather than arms on hips or folded.
- *Touch*: more touch in an appropriate manner.
- *Tone of voice*: higher pitch, upward contour, pure tone.
- *Verbal contents*: more self-disclosure.

The normal communication process is often presented as the information processing theory in the context of cognitive learning theory, which is discussed in Chapter 2.

## Generic and specialist communication skills

In addition to general communication skills, the mentor is likely to need to develop specialist communication skills to manage more complex mentee issues. Scammell (1990) suggests a communication continuum that spans generic communication at one end to specialist communication at the other, with the associated specific purposes and specific skills for each component on the continuum. These components and their associated purposes and skills are as follows:

| | |
|---|---|
| **Primary communications** | *purpose*: initial contacts with others; brief encounters<br>*skill*: simple interpersonal or social skills e.g. ability to listen, etc. |
| **Secondary communications** | *purpose*: ongoing relationships – verbal, non-verbal, written; informal support groups<br>*skill*: interpersonal or social skills, knowledge of how groups work, etc. |
| **Advice giving** | *purpose*: to offer factual information; to teach, instruct, supervise<br>*skill*: when to give advice, knowledge of subject, etc. |
| **Primary counselling** | *purpose*: support for friend or work colleague<br>*skill*: listen non-judgmentally, help with problem-solving, etc. |
| **Secondary counselling** | *purpose*: therapeutic counselling for specific mental health problems<br>*skill*: advanced accurate empathy, self-disclosure, etc. |

Primary and secondary communication occurs between mentor and mentee when exchanging information and establishing a working relationship. Beyond this level, the mentor may need to give direct advice to the student, especially when teaching, as well as when advice is requested. This, however, does not go as far as counselling, for which the individual requires more extensive training.

Primary counselling is a specialised communication skill that the mentor needs to develop to deal with difficult mentoring situations. Secondary counselling will be required for more intense psychological problems, which the mentor can deal with by directing the student to appropriate support services, or, if trained, by using a systematic approach such as Heron's (1989) six-category intervention analysis (see Box 1.3).

> ## Box 1.3   The six-category intervention analysis as a specialised communication skill
>
> ### Authoritative intervention
>
> - Prescriptive: giving advice
> - Informative: imparting information
> - Confrontational: directly challenging
>
> ### Facilitative intervention
>
> - Supportive: understanding and encouraging
> - Cathartic: allowing the release of emotions
> - Catalytic: encouraging deeper exploration

Heron's (1989) six-category intervention analysis therefore entails six possible actions that the counsellor can choose from. In difficult mentor–mentee situations, for every interaction, the mentor may decide which of the six categories is most appropriate. For instance, for a student who frequently claims to be feeling unwell, physically or psychologically, the mentor might use the prescriptive category of helping, and advise the mentee to consult the occupational health department. They might also give further information about where the department is, and the likely outcomes of this situation. In other situations, the mentor might use another one of the categories, for example cathartic, to enable the mentee to elaborate in detail how they feel about a patient whom they have looked after but who has passed away rather suddenly, for instance.

Another specialised communication skill involves communicating in one of three ways, or from one of three ego states (how we act, feel and behave) (Berne, 1975). It is known as transactional analysis and is illustrated in Figure 1.2.

In transactional analysis, every item of communication is uttered from one of the three ego states and received from one of the three ego states. Resolution of the interpersonal or psychological problem is achieved when both individuals communicate from adult ego states.

Transactional analysis is also a therapeutic technique that normally requires formal training. To extend communication skills to the arena of assessment of practice objectives, the mentor could find that they have to utilise specialised communication skills in helping and counselling the student who fails an assessment. This would entail aspects of counselling and helping skills that are relevant for the particular assessment situation, which is discussed in Chapter 7 of this book.

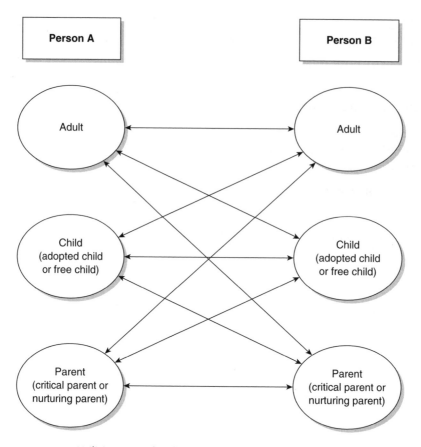

**FIGURE 1.2**    Utilising specialised communication skill: Transactional analysis

## Characteristics of mentors and enabling functions

### Activity 1.4    Characteristics of an effective mentor

Make a list of what you consider to be the characteristics of a registrant who is effective in their mentoring role for either pre- or post-registration students. Consider their characteristics from such perspectives as personal qualities, approach/actions and skills.

Responding to Activity 1.4 must have been straightforward as all healthcare professionals who have undertaken preparatory educational programmes that include practice placement will have encountered mentors. Some mentors may have been excellent, while there might have been reservations about others. Most of the characteristics identified by groups of student mentors are listed in Box 1.4.

---

### Box 1.4   Characteristics of the person who needs to act as mentor

- Patient
- Open-minded
- Approachable
- Have a good knowledge base
- Knowledge and competence is up to date
- Has good communication skills, including listening skills
- Provides encouragement
- Is self-motivated
- Shows concern, compassion, empathy
- Has teaching skills
- Provides psychological support
- Counsellor

- Tactful
- Diplomatic, fun and fair
- Willing to be a mentor
- Versatile, adaptable, flexible
- Allows time and commits self to it
- Confident
- Enthusiastic
- Advisor
- Is honest and trustworthy
- Trusting
- A role model
- Non-judgemental
- Resource facilitator
- Able to builder working relationship

---

In their study of students' perspectives on the qualities of the effective mentor, Gray and Smith (2000) list several characteristics, many of which are also identified in Box 1.4 above. At the final interview of this longitudinal three-year study, students identified 12 activities (akin to roles and responsibilities) that would make them good and effective mentors, including:

- Form a relaxed relationship with their student.
- Ascertain what the student requires as an individual to meet the desired learning outcomes.
- Think carefully about the duty rota in terms of arranging shifts to allow student and mentor to work together at some point each week.
- Allow the student some independence by giving more guidance at the beginning of the placement, then standing back and letting the student show initiative and self-motivation afterwards.

Darling (1984) reports on a study that explored various components of the mentor role. One of the most significant outcomes of the study was the identification of the characteristics of mentors that enable learning, which Darling identified as follows:

- **Role model** — Consciously practises nursing to a very high standard and conducts self in a way that the mentee can look to, value and adopt.

- **Energiser** — Is enthusiastic about the whole of nursing, inspires interest and motivates mentee.

- **Envisioner** — Is clear about how patient care could be even better, and is enthusiastic and dynamic about innovations.

- **Investor** — Invests an appropriate amount of time in the mentee, and imparts own knowledge and experience.

- **Supporter** — Encourages, gives time, is always willing to listen and makes himself or herself available in times of need.

- **Standard prodder** — Always questioning standards of care and competence and is clear about own standards.

- **Teacher-coach** — Teaches patient care-related knowledge and competence skilfully, gives guidance, allows time to practise and encourages the student to learn through experience.

- **Feedback giver** — Provides positive feedback, points out weaknesses and discusses further learning.

- **Eye opener** — Inspires interest in wider issues, political, financial, etc., and departmental initiatives that can impact on the practice setting or specialism.

- **Door opener** — Suggests available healthcare provisions and learning opportunities related to practice objectives.

- **Ideas bouncer** — Encourages mentee to generate and verbalise new ideas, listens to them and helps mentee to reflect on them.

- **Problem solver** — Helps the mentee to think systematically about problems and ways of resolving and preventing them.

- **Career counsellor** — Available to offer own views and guidance in career planning.

- **Challenger** — Enables the mentee to think more critically about their decisions, and challenges views, opinions and beliefs.

Each mentor characteristic can be explored in detail as a concept in its own right, and to illustrate this, the next section explores the characteristic of 'role model' and then of 'challenger and supporter'.

## The mentor as the role model

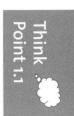

### A role model

Consider the terms *model* and *modelling*. Next, consider what a role model is. Consider also why healthcare professionals need to be role models, who for, and what it is about a person that makes him or her a role model.

In response to Think Point 1.1, you might have felt that a mentor who is a role model is someone who fulfils NMC's (2008a) standards for mentors, as identified earlier in this chapter. Although the mentor would be a role model predominantly for clinical skills, they should also be a role model as an organiser of care, a researcher and a teacher within the parameters of their post.

As with most nascent and tentative concepts, a concept analysis or a STEP (social, technical, economic and political) analysis can enable further clarification of the concept, and a systematic understanding of various facets and components of the concept. Alternatively, a SWOT (strengths, weaknesses, opportunities and threats) analysis can be undertaken. Such an analysis can help the individual decide whether any problem-solving, avoidance or developmental actions need to be taken.

### Activity 1.5   STEP analysis of role model

Using the headings social, technical, economic and political, conduct a STEP analysis of 'the mentor as a role model'.

Being a role model is a feature of Bandura's (1997) social learning theory, which stipulates that substantial learning occurs as a result of observation of appropriate professionals. Bahn (2001) suggests that role modelling is consistent with social learning theory, as substantial socialisation occurs in clinical learning environments. It is also a significant component of 'work-based learning', which is discussed in Chapter 4.

There can also be bad role models, that is, how not to come over as a healthcare professional. Bad role models can therefore not be seen as a model at all, considering what the word 'model' means. A role model is 'an exemplary person or thing, a perfect exemplar of excellence' (Brown, 2002: 1806), that is, someone whose practice standards, attitudes and beliefs the observer can emulate. Individuals choose their role models, such as someone who is good at time management, at self-organisation, or in how they interact with colleagues.

Donaldson and Carter (2005) report on an evaluation of the perceptions of undergraduate students on role modelling within the clinical learning environment. They indicate that students stressed the importance of good role models whose competence they could observe and practise. Constructive feedback was needed on their practice from their role models to develop their competence and build up their confidence, and to convert observed behaviour into their own behaviour and skill set.

Thomas (2005) reports that there are mixed views about nurses being role models of healthy habits when off duty. Faugier (2005a) suggests that role models are those whom we look up to, emulate and admire as professionals. However, in society in general, she suggests, people base their character identities, values and lifestyles on celebrities and characters in television programmes. This highlights how crucial the latter's public behaviours are. All teachers in the practice setting (e.g. mentors) should therefore be aware of their impact as role models on students' learning of skills and professional attitudes.

### The mentor as a challenger and supporter

There are various examples of situations that present high or low challenge for learners in practice settings, and the support required. Asking a third-year student nurse consistently to perform clinical skills for which they have already been signed as competent would provide a lesser challenge to them, and lesser support might be required. But if the same student hasn't yet learnt how to provide care in epidural pain control, for instance, then this would present a higher challenge and the student is likely to need a high level of support.

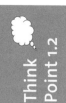

**Think Point 1.2**

## Mentoring support and challenge

Consider the characteristics of 'supporter' and 'challenger' identified by Darling (1984) and think of learning situations where you need to provide the mentee with a high level of challenge and support, and other situations where you afford low levels of each.

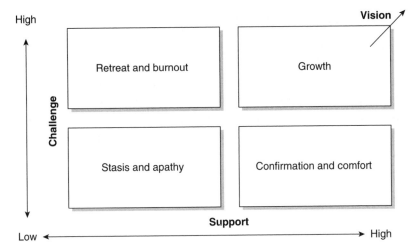

**FIGURE 1.3**   Effects of support and challenge on the mentee's development

Daloz (1989) explored these two functions further and concluded that high support and challenge can lead to growth and achievement of vision, while low support and low challenge can result in stasis and apathy, as illustrated in Figure 1.3.

---

## Activity 1.6   Ascertaining mentorship potential

Consider Darling's (1984) characteristics or roles of the mentor as detailed in Box 1.5, and identify situations where you needed to use these skills in relation to mentoring learners or of forthcoming opportunities for mentoring.

1   For each characteristic, do a self-rating of yourself as a mentor using numbers 1 to 4, 1 indicating development or learning need and 4 indicating skilled.
2   Next, focus on one or two of the skills on which you rate yourself as low, and consider why this is (e.g. lack of opportunity) and how you can develop this characteristic.

---

The above exercise based on characteristics or roles of the mentor is also referred to as 'measuring mentorship potential' (MMP) (Darling, 1984). The characteristics or attributes of the effective preceptor, on the other hand, were identified earlier in this chapter.

## Mentor actions to support learning

The roles and responsibilities of the effective mentor are regularly researched to ascertain the more contemporary nature and perceptions of this function. For example, Carnwell et al. (2007) explored NHS and HEI managers' perceptions of learning support roles, and found that the mentors' primary role is in clinical practice, their primary skills constituting clinical expertise, teaching clinical skills and student support, and their primary focus being the individual student, that is student supervision and assessment of students' clinical skills. However, they also identified potential for role conflict, particularly if the mentor is relatively recently qualified, and therefore still developing their own repertoire of clinical skills.

Taking a broader perspective, Hall et al. (2008) explored mentors' perceptions of the role in teacher training in the USA, and found that it comprises being:

- parent figure
- trouble shooter
- scaffolder
- counsellor
- supporter
- instructional model
- coach or guide
- source of advice
- a sounding board for concerns about teaching

Of course, the teacher mentor has to be a role model in teaching in the first place, and in healthcare the mentor has to be a role model as a healthcare professional, i.e. as a clinician as well.

---

## Activity 1.7   Actions that support learning

In addition to having the characteristics of an effective mentor (e.g. Box 1.5), think of and make a list of a number of actions that can be taken by mentors that support learning.

---

No doubt a range of components that support learning can be identified. One of the key functions of the mentor is to help the student integrate into the practice setting, which entails managing the practice placement, receiving the student and conducting initial, mid-placement and final interviews, and possibly using learning contracts. Acceptance of the mentee (Rogers and

Freiberg, 1994) signifies that the mentor accepts the student for their current levels of knowledge and competence, which may be extensive or minimal.

As for managing the placement, the designated mentor would have been nominated before the student, starts on the placement and would need self-preparation time beforehand. Time would also have been set aside for receiving the student and introducing them to the team, and associate mentors would have been identified.

Seeing the practice placement from a student's viewpoint suggests that they might be experiencing different feelings in anticipation of the placement. They are likely to appreciate any prior information sent to them, which might include any preparatory reading that the student can do. On the first day, they tend to appreciate an introduction to the clinical area, making them feel comfortable about learning, a professional but friendly environment, student involvement and continuity of mentorship. These perspectives are consistent with 'empathic understanding' identified as a key condition of effective working relationships by Rogers and Freiberg (1994).

Furthermore, the NMC (2008a) indicates that to enable effective learning, at least 40 per cent of the student's placement time must be spent working with the mentor. Similar rules apply to the practice teacher role. Moreover, the NMC (e.g. 2008a) has identified the need for 'protected time' for mentoring as has the Department of Health (1999). Mentoring can be made even more efficient by the use of learning contracts.

## Using learning contracts

Learning contracts are very much a feature of adult education (or andragogy, which is discussed in Chapter 2) and involve negotiated learning between teacher and student. As the word *contract* implies, a learning contract is a written and signed agreement between teacher (mentor in this case) and learner resulting in the latter's active involvement in decisions over practice objectives and other components of learning. Therefore, it is often a feature of practice modules whereby the mentor and student agree on specific practice objectives and on each party's responsibility in the achievement of the objectives.

The use of learning contracts was advocated by Knowles et al. (1998) in the context of adult learners needing to exercise some self-direction in their learning. The agreed set of objectives in the learning contract includes those of the course curriculum and those of the student and the mentor. Therefore, the learning contract affords the student some control over their learning, motivates them to learn and to engage with the placement experience. It is also a medium for identifying the student's pace of learning, to explore the means of theory and practice integration, and can be supported by ascertaining the student's preferred learning style.

However, the requirements and objectives set by the course curriculum have to be met. A learning contract section or pro forma may already have been included in the student's placement competencies booklet. Basically, the mentor and student discuss and agree on what the student is aiming to learn, how the learning will take place and how this will be evaluated. This is usually written down by the student and, when agreed, both mentor and student sign and date it. Learning pathways based on patient journeys can be incorporated as a strategy for achieving particular objectives. An example of a learning contract is presented in Box 1.5.

## Box 1.5    A learning contract

| Name of student: | | | Cohort: | |
|---|---|---|---|---|
| Placement: | | | Mentor's name: | |
| *Learning needs* | *Objectives* | *Resource and strategies* | *Target date* | *Evidence* |
| What do I want to learn? – Topic area | What do I want to have achieved at the end of this learning? – Specific objectives | How will I learn, and who will support me? – Learning strategies | Date of achieving the objectives | How will I know I have achieved my intended learning? |
| Assessment of a new patient | Able to assess the health and social care needs of newly admitted/ referred patient / service user | Mentor, social worker | 30–09– 2010 | Mentor reviews and agrees with my assessment and care plan |

*(Continued)*

*(Continued)*

| Teach patients | Able to teach a type 2 diabetic patient how to control their dietary intake | Mentor, dietician. Consult diet sheets, guidelines. Read up on type 2 diabetes | 30–09–2010 | Mentor observes my teaching and signs me as competent in this skill |
|---|---|---|---|---|
| Pre-contract | | | | |

| Signature of student: | Date: |
|---|---|

| Mentor's signature: | Date: |
|---|---|

| Name of link teacher / practice education facilitator: | Name of personal tutor: |
|---|---|

| Comments on achievement of contract objectives | |
|---|---|

| Signature of student: | Date: |
|---|---|

| Mentor's signature: | Date: |
|---|---|

Crucial components of the learning contract are also the specific resources (human and material) that are required to enable the student to achieve the agreed objectives, and also the specific dates by which each objective will have been achieved. An alternative to a learning contract is a learning agreement (Open University, 2001; RCN, 2002), which has similar features but might not include signatures of those involved, nor rigid 'achieve-by' dates.

## The learning contract

What would logically happen after both parties have signed the learning contract? Do you feel that it should be constantly reviewed to monitor the student's progress with its content, or only reviewed on the 'target date'?

Learning contracts may be seen by some as a chore. Others may prefer to write something treating it as a mere formality. But the benefits of learning contracts have been reported by Ghazi and Henshaw (1998), for instance, who found that learning contracts help to improve student performance in assessments and student attendance at lectures. Donaldson (1992), Northcott (1989) and others reported similar benefits.

An important step involved in constructing a learning contract is the mentor facilitating self-assessment of clinical skills and knowledge by the student and identifying inherent learning needs. Naturally, when a contract has been drawn up, then on the 'achieve-by' date there will be a need to ascertain whether the activities identified in the contract were undertaken and the objectives achieved. The review time will of course have been determined at the beginning when the content was being discussed and documented.

The mentor will have developed knowledge and understanding on the use of learning contracts as part of the mentor preparation programme, along with how they can deliver these functions in the context of other roles that they have to fulfil.

Rogers and Freiberg (1994) indicate that learning contracts endow the student some freedom to learn aspects that they wish to learn and pursue areas that they find particularly interesting. A learning contract is also a medium for resolving any doubt that there may be about specific purposes of the learning experience. It clarifies the activities that the student would engage in and provides motivation and reinforcement through the achievement of objectives.

Having determined that a contract can be a very useful educational tool, no doubt you'll be wondering what happens if the student does not take all the actions that they had agreed to take or does not achieve all the specified objectives.

There are mixed views in the literature about whether learning contracts are legally binding. Mazhindu (1990) argues that they are, while Neary (2000a) suggests that this isn't the case. It is useful to note the NMC's (2009c) stance on documentation and record keeping as it indicates that written as well as electronically kept records comprise evidence of actions taken (or omitted). For learning contracts to be effective, they need to be skilfully constructed. Guidelines for constructing them are provided by educational researchers Knowles et al. (1998), as well as by Bailey and Tuohy (2009) more recently, and an example of a well-constructed learning contract is presented in Box 1.6 above.

## Adverse Effects of Poor Mentoring

A common experience in nursing in the twenty-first century is that nurses working in many practice settings feel that they are managing their workload with ongoing staffing constraints. Indeed, Phillips et al. (2000) noted that mentors fulfil their mentoring role as one of several other roles they have during any span of duty. Despite 'protected time' for mentoring having been advocated for over a decade (DH, 1999; NMC, 2008a), the implementation of this mechanism remains slow for many mentors due to the demands on their time. When working within these constraints, knowingly or unknowingly, the mentor may be taking actions that discourage learning.

### Activity 1.8   How the mentor might discourage learning

Think of, and make notes on, a range of actions on the part of mentors that, advertently or inadvertently, may be seen as discouraging or disabling learning.

The following case study presents an example of poor mentoring.

## 🗁 Case Study – Poor mentoring

Mel Alexis is a second-year student nurse on a rehabilitation ward. One day, she finished her shift early, having told the staff nurse in charge that she had a terrible headache, while in fact she was extremely upset regarding her placement.

That morning she had felt that the staff nurse had spoken to her in a very unprofessional manner, as she does to patients as well. This is what bothered Mel the most. She also challenged the staff nurse over her drug administration that morning. A patient was left her morning medication in a pot on the table, but was unable to swallow it as she needed assistance due to her having a weak side and problems with her other hand. As Mel walked past the patient's room, the patient called her and indicated that she had not taken her tablets yet. As Mel was not the nurse who administered the drugs, she called the nurse to the room for her to administer the drugs. The nurse said that she did not have time to do this but the tablets were correct for the patient.

Mel agreed to assist in giving the medication but noticed three tablets lying on the table beside the pot. Mel asked the nurse what these tablets were and she was advised they were morning medications as well. Mel doubted this as they were not in the medicine pot and asked the nurse why they were not in the pot, but the latter did not give an answer and instead picked them up and put them into the pot. The nurse then told Mel to assist with the medications and Mel made it clear that she did not feel that the medications were correct, as there seemed to be more tablets than the patient usually took in the morning. The nurse told Mel not to question her drug administration, so Mel felt that she had no choice but to assist the patient in taking the drugs.

This event highlighted Mel's unhappiness with this ward. She had started feeling like this on day one when she was not introduced to any staff members or shown around.

She had had to find things out for herself during her time on this ward and if she asked where something was, the staff said it would be quicker for them to get the item themselves rather than show Mel. As a second-year nurse, she was expecting to do many nursing activities but instead she felt that she was being treated like a support worker. Although Mel loves providing basic nursing care to patients, she expected a lot more out of this placement than she was actually achieving. Mel appreciates that on a rehabilitation ward nursing takes on a different role but she feels that she has yet to see what this role is.

Mel says she has always wanted to be a nurse and really loves the job, but this ward has now made her question this and it makes her very sad to feel like this.

In response to Activity 1.8, you may have felt that one of the problems that students experience is the lack of opportunities to work with their named mentor. Other actions on the part of mentors that you might have thought of that can discourage learning are:

- lack of interest in students and in their learning needs;
- lack of knowledge about the student's course;
- lack of evidence-based practice or research utilisation;
- hierarchical, and a lack of team approach;
- not acknowledging student's previous experience;
- negative attitudes;
- reluctant to change practice.

There is a possibility that you have yourself witnessed poor mentoring, directly or indirectly. Other problems with mentoring remain prevalent. Earlier research into mentoring and assessing had identified personality characteristics that discourage learning. For instance, Darling's (1985) qualitative study revealed what she termed the characteristics of the 'galaxy of toxic mentors' (see Box 1.6).

---

### Box 1.6 The 'galaxy of toxic mentors'

| Types | Features |
| --- | --- |
| Avoiders | Mentors who are not available or accessible, also referred to as ignorers or non-responders. |
| Dumpers | Throw people into new roles or situations and let them flounder, either to sink or to swim, often deliberately. |
| Blockers | Actively avoid meeting the mentee's needs either by refusing requests, by controlling through withholding information, or by blocking the mentee's development by over-supervising. |
| Destroyers/ Criticisers | Set out to destroy the mentee by subtle attacks to undermine confidence, and open and public verbal attacks and arguments, questioning of abilities and deliberately destroying confidence. |

Based on extensive experience in management and the processes of decision-making, Heirs and Farrell (1986) explored the mindsets of individual employees who enable an organisation to progress with its aims, and those of people who block this development. While the focus is on looking for, and developing, 'talents' in employees, the reality is that the mindset of some individuals can stifle development. These authors grouped the problematic or disabling traits, termed 'three mental poisons', as the functioning of rigid minds, ego minds and Machiavellian minds (see Box 1.7). Such ways of thinking are not always obvious, nor easily detected, but do affect learning adversely.

---

## Box 1.7   The functioning of rigid minds, ego minds and Machiavellian minds

### The rigid mind:

- Personal values are set or stereotyped
- Unable to see the positiveness in others' thoughts if they conflict with their thinking
- Continually blocks the openness of more creative thinking
- Loyal to traditional thinking and rejects novelty (seen as complexity)
- Appears to lack imagination or creativity
- Stifles use of originality and encourages complacency

### The ego mind:

- Sees elements of a problem only in terms of self-interest and self-importance
- Fairly ambitious and has a high opinion of own abilities
- Looks after number one to the exclusion of other considerations
- Pays little attention to what others think and say
- Unsociable and do not contribute to collective thinking, will betray colleagues and even the organisation if it serves his or her ends

### The Machiavellian mind:

- Quickly sees the range of likely outcomes of any decision
- Manipulates the feelings and ambitions of others to deceive
- Devious and calculating
- Intimidates and engages in politicking
- Perpetuates worry in the organisation and perpetually currying favour with superiors
- Scheming, cunning and suspicious of subordinates

*Source*: Heirs and Farrell (1986)

Mentoring was formalised with increased emphasis with the introduction of Diploma in higher education programmes in Nursing (Project 2000) (UKCC, 1999), and in this context, Gray and Smith (2000) conducted a study to explore students' experiences of mentoring, and found that whilst effective and good mentoring did prevail, the majority of students also experienced poor mentoring, as some mentors:

- Break promises
- Lack knowledge and expertise
- Have poor teaching skills
- Have no structure to their teaching
- 'Chop and change their minds'
- Allow students to observe only (i.e. not participate)
- Are unclear about their students' capabilities
- Throw students in at the deep end
- Delegate unwanted jobs to students
- Dislike their job and/or students
- May be disliked by other members of the team
- Are distant, less friendly, unapproachable
- Intimidate the students
- Have unrealistic expectations

---

## Activity 1.9    Mentors who disable learning

Discuss with a peer or in a small group why any mentor would behave in the negative ways described by Darling or Gray and Smith. Discuss also if and how such behaviours can be changed.

---

Darling (1985) makes a number of suggestions on how to deal with toxic mentors. For instance, if the particular mentor–mentee allocation is unavoidable, then the mentee can try and keep the relationship balanced by building a support network with other students or registrants within the team, and drawing on his or her own personal strengths (e.g. problem-solving skills). Heirs and Farrell (1986) suggest that it is the organisation's managers' responsibility to identify individuals who fall into any of these categories. Their 'poisonous' thinking endures, but can be changed gradually through formal and informal meetings. Decisions about delegation of responsibilities and roles need to be applied selectively.

Other actions that can be taken if ineffective mentoring is detected is to implement co-mentoring, which involves two mentors jointly mentoring the student. A temporary non-allocation of a mentee to the ineffective mentor is another alternative that might work. Managers can formally or informally ask the mentor how well they feel they are fulfilling their mentoring role. The line manager may be able to confront the ineffective mentor if poor mentoring has been observed, or a complaint received. There can be alternative strategies which are dependent on local circumstances. Ethical aspects of poor mentoring are discussed in Chapter 7.

## Approaches and Models of Effective Mentoring

Despite the multiplicity of likely mentor behaviours that could inhibit learning, mentoring remains a necessary role for supporting learning in healthcare professions. A mentor in personal life is also advocated. Due to the humane, personal and suffering-prevention nature of healthcare provision, professional education programmes need to be appropriately structured and carefully monitored. Mentoring students must also be a structured or planned exercise, as discussed earlier in this chapter. An appropriate combination of directive and facilitative approaches may be adopted, depending on the knowledge and competence the student displays.

The underlying principles on which each mentor bases their mentoring vary according to the personal beliefs and approaches of the mentor towards this role. The underpinning beliefs of the mentor about student learning therefore determine their approach to mentoring, and the model or framework of mentoring they use.

The differences between the terms *approach, model* and *framework* are as follows. Approach to mentoring is personal to the mentor, and is based on his or her own life and professional experiences, personal views and beliefs. In mentoring, it would depend on the mentor's beliefs about nursing, pre-registration course design, student and learner populations and their styles of learning.

A model, however, can be defined as a research-deduced, and therefore informed, set of interrelated components that enable the activity to be addressed comprehensively. A framework takes this further, whereupon the components of the model are utilised as sections or headings for planning and implementing the activity, and may even have been empirically tested.

All three perspectives indicate a planned and systematic approach to the mentee's placement experience to make it more effective. Few frameworks for mentoring in healthcare are currently available. Darling's (1984) roles or characteristics of the mentor constitute such a model, the NMC's (2008a) eight domain standards for mentoring is another. Despite the pragmatic nature of frameworks, it is important to examine other approaches and models of mentoring that are available, such as those identified in Box 1.8.

## Box 1.8 Approaches, models and frameworks for mentoring

### Approaches to mentoring

| | |
|---|---|
| Classical mentoring | Also known as informal or primary mentoring. A natural, mutual and self-chosen relationship that can usually be terminated by mutual decision. |
| Reflective practitioner | Based on learning theories, e.g. andragogy, styles of learning and student-centred approaches, the mentor is a critical friend and co-enquirer. |

### Models or frameworks of mentoring

| | |
|---|---|
| Apprenticeship model | The mentor as skilled crafts person, and the mentee learns by re-enacting their actions. |
| Competence-based model | The mentor enables the mentee to learn specific practice objectives, and assesses their competence in them. |
| Team mentoring model | A team of mentors mentor one or more students jointly, as recommended for nursing by Phillips et al. (2000), for instance. Is akin to team supervision for doctorate students. |
| Contract mentoring | Formal mentoring that is time- or objectives-restricted, e.g. when on practice placement at another institution. |
| Pseudo-mentoring | Also known as quasi- or partial mentoring, may be in appearance only, and for a specific task, e.g. dissertation supervision. |

A model is of course useful if it can be used as a framework for action. Kerry and Mayes (1995) tend to use the terms 'strategies', 'approaches' and 'models' interchangeably. They suggest four models of mentoring, namely the:

- Colleagual model – similar to team mentoring or the use of associate mentors.
- Counselling model – refers to facilitation of learning using humanistic theories (discussed in Chapter 2).
- Professional model – similar to the contract model, for example for a student on a practice placement, or in dissertation supervision (i.e. for a specific task).
- Process model – also referring to facilitation of learning but enabling the mentee eventually to become an independent practitioner.

## Activity 1.10   Application of models of mentoring

In your own experience of mentorship, which of these approaches, models or frameworks apply to learning professional skills in your own practice setting, and why? Which ones suit you most? Make some notes.

It could be argued that often the apprenticeship model applies more to the training of support workers in that an apprentice normally learns skills and crafts at the level of task performance, along with associated practical knowledge, unlike the holistic psycho-bio-social approach taken by nurses and midwives. The competence model might apply to nursing but the reader needs to be aware of varying definitions of the term *competence*. Some definitions see competence as the ability to perform a skill in accordance with agreed procedures and incorporate practical knowledge, while others see it as including theoretical knowledge as well.

The reflective practitioner approach is one that is frequently favoured within health profession circles, and advocates the mentor taking a less directive approach to their practice-based teaching. Consider the following reflective recording in the portfolio of a student social worker – Sheila.

## Case Study – Sheila's portfolio

I visited Mr J while his care co-ordinator, who is also my practice supervisor, was on annual leave. At this time he expressed concern about his care co-ordinator and questioned her supportive abilities. My initial reaction was to explain that different practitioners would use different approaches, and advised him to raise the issue with the care co-ordinator. In a further conversation by telephone, Mr J reiterated the issue but in a more agitated manner and asked me to speak to the care co-ordinator. His care co-ordinator suggested that we visit Mr J to question him about what he actually wanted from the service and what type of support he felt she should offer. She felt Mr J didn't always engage with services (he frequently missed appointments), and that his drug-addiction problem was the issue he most needed to address, but which she did not specialise in. Mr J was receiving services from the drug team but, again, he didn't always attend his appointments. However, it was clear Mr J felt he

*(Continued)*

*(Continued)*

needed more support. As a result we discussed a referral to an agency which provided outreach support specifically for people with a history of offending and drug/alcohol abuse problems. Mr J was keen to accept this support.

Reflective recordings from clinical situations provide an essential learning vehicle for mentees. The approaches and models presented in Box 1.9 may not all be seen as frameworks although they can be systematic and comprehensive. Most of the approaches are relatively recent concepts that await further empirical exploration or testing. Other frameworks and models of good practice are identified as specific sets of actions for specific professions, such as in business mentoring (Institute of Directors, 2010). The RCN (2002) presents them as the 'responsibilities' of mentors.

## Further dimensions of mentoring

To enable healthcare professionals to fulfil their mentor role effectively, especially towards students on pre-qualifying education programmes, they are required to undergo specified educational preparation. They thus have to attend, and successfully complete an NMC-approved mentor course. One requirement for such courses is that they address the theory and practice related to the mentor outcomes under the eight NMC (2008a) domains referred to earlier in this chapter.

Fulton et al. (2007) explored the international literature for the content of mentor programmes, and concluded that although the NMC domains (they were originally published in 2006) provide an acceptable framework for mentoring, it is reasonable to expect each country to be able to adapt the framework according to their own national and local needs.

The NMC (2008a) indicates that educational preparation for mentors need to be at a minimum academic level 5 (Quality Assurance Agency for Higher Education (QAA), 2008), although most of these programmes are at degree and postgraduate levels (levels 6 and 7 (QAA, 2008), respectively). They tend to be equivalent to 200 to 300 hours of student effort, and are normally completed within four months. Continuing learning for mentors subsequent to successful completion of a mentor preparation programme is discussed in Chapter 8.

Furthermore, as noted earlier in this chapter, mentoring is now an activity that is widely applied in various healthcare and non-healthcare fields, and can take different forms. Previously, mentoring in nursing, and currently in medicine (GMC, 2010), comprised mentors and mentees being mutually selected for their respective roles by the two healthcare professionals for facilitation, guidance, assistance and support with student learning. The notion that students can select their mentor has currency in some situations, such as if the named mentor's job changes at short notice.

Gilmour et al. (2007) report on a highly successful peer-mentoring programme in which second-year student nurses mentor first-year students as they embark on their pre-registration university courses. Furthermore, a small-scale study by van Eps et al. (2006) suggests that year-long mentorship programmes yield more beneficial outcomes for students in terms of the variety of skills that they acquire through the longer-term relationship than other ones.

Long-arm mentoring is another activity that tends to prevail primarily in certain areas of primary and social care where the mentor is not generally based on the same healthcare site as the mentee, and yet all criteria and activities comprising effective mentoring are fulfilled. Electronic or e-mentoring can also be implemented successfully, as demonstrated by Stewart and Carpenter (2009), whereupon the mentor and the mentee communicate entirely through their computers.

However, in a study of students' experiences and staff perceptions of the implementation of placement development teams, Williamson (2009) reports that students indicate a need for more direct, personal and organisational support, and better communication between university and placement areas. Furthermore, research also suggests that the effectiveness of the mentor role also depends on the level of the mentor's interest in mentoring (e.g. Hallin and Danielson, 2009).

## Chapter Summary

This chapter has focused on mentoring as a concept and professional role, and has therefore addressed:

- Current and recent perspectives on the concept mentoring, definitions of and distinctions between the mentor's and various related learning facilitation roles, such as preceptors, clinical educators, assessors and supervisors, and those of the practice education facilitator, link tutor and personal tutor. All these roles are established to facilitate healthcare learners acquire clinical skills, knowledge and appropriate attitudes.
- A number of reasons for requiring mentors for supporting learning for healthcare students on preparatory education programmes during practice placements, and the criteria for who can be a mentor.

- Effective mentoring, which encompasses effective working relationships, relevant mentor–mentee communication, and includes generic and specialist communication skills; the characteristics of mentors and enabling functions, which include the mentor as a role model for learners, and ascertaining own mentorship potential; the actions that support learning including the use of learning contracts.
- Research findings on detrimental effects of poor, inefficient or adverse mentoring.
- The use of different models or approaches that identify mentors' perceptions of their mentoring role.

# Further Optional Reading

For an exploration of research on mentoring and coaching in a wide range of settings in the UK and abroad, and discussion on a range of perspectives and issues, see:

- Garvey, B., Stokes, P. and Megginson, D. (2009) *Coaching and Mentoring: Theory and Practice*. London: SAGE.

For management mentoring and other models of mentoring, see:

- Megginson, D., Clutterbuck, D., Garvey, B., Stokes, P. and Garrett-Harris, R. (2006) *Mentoring in Action: A Practical Guide*. London: Kogan Page.

For three very recent articles on clinical supervision, see:

- Waskett, C. (2010) 'Clinical supervision using the 4S model 1: Considering the structure and setting it up', *Nursing Times,* 106 (16): 12–14.

To explore original directives and guidelines related to effective mentoring and supervision see also the health and social care regulatory bodies' (e.g. HPC, GSCC) and professional colleges' (e.g. RCN, COT) websites, such as that of the Chartered Society of Physiotherapy's (2004) *Accreditation of Clinical Educators (ACE)* publication which provides an update on the scheme and the number of physiotherapists who had been accredited through the scheme.

- Charted Society of Physiotherapy (2004) *Accreditation of Clinical Educators Scheme*. Available at: www.csp.org.uk/uploads/documents/csp_ace_scheme_guidance.pdf. Accessed 4 August 2010.

For details of the link between *NHS KSF* (DH, 2004a) dimensions and indicators for band 5 healthcare staff and precepteeship, see:

- College of Occupational Therapists (2006) *The Preceptorship Training Manual – A Resource for Occupational Therapists*. London: COT.

For details of successful implementation of preceptorship, see:

- Scottish Government (2010) *Flying Start NHS*. Available at: http://flyingstart.scot.nhs. uk/. Accessed 20 December 2010.

As preceptorship is being implemented with renewed vigour, it should prove advanta-geous for you to arrange to meet the main trust-based preceptorship co-ordinator to ascertain their perspective on this enterprise, i.e. their specific plans for implementation, and for dealing with anticipated and unanticipated issues.

For a discussion on the ten most commonly utilised models of practice education roles, essentially reflecting different learning facilitation and student roles, e.g. joint appointments, internship, etc., see:

- Budgen, C. and Gamroth, L. (2008) 'An overview of practice education models', *Nurse Education Today*, 28 (3): 273–83.

For a good section on vicarious learning, see pp. 86–101 of:

- Bandura, A. (1997) *Self-Efficacy – The Exercise of Control*. New York: W H Freeman and Company.

# 2
# How Learners Learn

## Introduction

As patient or service user care interventions are the main part of healthcare professionals' work, an appropriate proportion of their pre-registration education courses are dedicated to developing students' clinical and psycho-social care skills. In the nursing pre-registration course, for instance, which amounts to a total of 4600 hours of learning in three years, the NMC (2010a) requires a minimum of 50 per cent of this learning time to be utilised in learning patient or service user care skills mostly in practice settings. Learning in practice settings therefore occupies a pivotal role in pre-registration education. Indeed, learning is an ongoing requirement for all healthcare professionals throughout their careers.

Consequently, this chapter and Chapter 3 are based on 'facilitation of learning', which is also one of the eight domains in the NMC's (2008a: 51) standards for supporting learning, and under this domain the NMC indicates that mentors must 'facilitate learning for a range of students, within a particular area of practice where appropriate, encouraging self-management of learning opportunities and providing support to maximise individual potential'. The outcomes for mentors under this domain are:

- use knowledge of the student's stage of learning to select appropriate learning opportunities to meet individual needs;
- facilitate the selection of appropriate learning strategies to integrate learning from practice and academic experiences;
- support students in critically reflecting upon their learning experiences in order to enhance future learning.

Chapter 2 draws on multiple theories of learning and focuses on ways in which healthcare professionals learn the competence and knowledge required for patient or service user care delivery. Ways in which the mentor facilitates learning is examined in Chapter 3, and how practice settings can also be effective learning environments, in Chapter 4.

## Chapter outcomes

On completion of this chapter, you should be able to:

1   Identify the specific knowledge and competence that learners and healthcare profession students learn during their pre-registration education programmes, including different types of knowledge and professional skills.
2   Identify various reasons for learning by different individuals, and the nature of professional competence.
3   Analyse prevailing major views and perspectives on learning, teaching and education.
4   Understand and critically analyse key theories of learning, and indicate how they can be applied to learning in practice settings.
5   Comprehend the different styles and approaches to learning, and ways in which mentors can adapt their style of teaching to mentees' individual learning styles and approaches.

# What do Healthcare Learners Learn, and Why?

The first section of this chapter begins by identifying the specific knowledge and competencies that learners in healthcare professions learn, in particular during their initial preparatory programmes.

## Healthcare competencies

For nurse education programmes, the NMC (2010a) identifies the competencies that students have to achieve to gain the Registered Nurse (RN) qualification. The NMC's (2010a) standards for pre-registration education are being implemented from 2011 (and from 2013 by all HEIs offering pre-registration nurse education programmes). Education programmes prior to those based on the NMC (2010a) standards are based on the NMC (2004a) 'Standards of Proficiency' (SOP) in which the competencies to be achieved in the common foundation programme and branch programmes are identified under the four domains: (i) professional and ethical practice, (ii) care delivery, (iii) care management, and (iv) personal and professional development.

In its 'competency framework', the NMC (2010a) standards identify first, 'generic competencies' that student nurses in all four 'fields' of practice (previously referred to as branch) must achieve during their education programme, the four fields being:

- adult nursing
- mental health nursing
- learning disabilities nursing
- children's nursing

Second, the standards identify the generic, as well as a set of field-specific competencies for each of the four fields under the following four domains:

- professional values
- communication and interpersonal skills
- nursing practice and decision-making
- leadership, management and teamworking

As can be expected, the NMC provides comprehensive details of all areas of competence that students must achieve to be able to have their name entered on the NMC's register as a 'registrant' in the particular field of practice. Under the domain 'Nursing practice and decision-making', for instance, it identifies the generic competencies as well as ten field-specific competencies – a few examples of field competencies under this domain for 'adult nurses' are reproduced in Box 2.1.

---

**Box 2.1    Field standard of competence for adult nurses under the domain 'Nursing practice and decision-making'**

All nurses must use up-to-date knowledge and evidence to assess, plan, deliver and evaluate care, communicate findings, influence change and promote health and best practice. They must make person-centred, evidence-based judgements and decisions, in partnership with others involved in the care process, to ensure high quality care. They must be able to recognise when the complexity of clinical decisions requires specialist knowledge and expertise, and consult or refer accordingly.

1   **Adult nurses** must be able to recognise and respond to the needs of all people who come into their care including babies, children and young people, pregnant and postnatal women, people with mental health problems, people with physical disabilities, people with learning disabilities, older people, and people with long term problems such as cognitive impairment.

*(Continued)*

*(Continued)*

2   All nurses must possess a broad knowledge of the structure and functions of the human body, and other relevant knowledge from the life, behavioural and social sciences as applied to health, ill health, disability, ageing and death. They must have an in-depth knowledge of common physical and mental health problems and treatments in their own field of practice, including co-morbidity and physiological and psychological vulnerability.

3   All nurses must carry out comprehensive, systematic nursing assessments that take account of relevant physical, social, cultural, psychological, spiritual, genetic and environmental factors, in partnership with service users and others through interaction, observation and measurement.

4   **Adult nurses** must safely use a range of diagnostic skills, employing appropriate technology, to assess the needs of service users.

5   All nurses must ascertain and respond to the physical, social and psychological needs of people, groups and communities. They must then plan, deliver and evaluate safe, competent, person-centred care in partnership ....

*Source*: NMC (2010a: 17–18)

As can be seen in Box 2.1, there are also sub–competencies identified under some of the competencies. No doubt it should prove useful for all mentors to have access to a hard copy of the whole *Standards for Pre-registration Nursing Education* (NMC, 2010a) document to refer to as and when required.

The NMC undertook a number of public and professional consultations to arrive at the content of the pre-registration nurse education programme, one of the highlights of which has been the decision to include 'essential skills clusters' (ESCs) within these programmes. It indicates that the ESCs should be incorporated into all pre-registration nursing programmes as they can be used to develop learning outcomes at different levels, they can be mapped to specific competencies within the domains, and also used for developing practice assessment frameworks (NMC, 2010a). It also indicates that all ESCs apply to all fields of nursing, and they can support the achievement of set competencies and criteria, which can be demonstrated on assessment of competence at specific progression points.

Forty-two areas of competencies are identified under the five clusters: (i) care, compassion and communication; (ii) organisational aspects of care; (iii) infection prevention and control; (iv) nutrition and fluid management;

and (v) medicines management. Students have to demonstrate competence in each of the skills under the 42 areas of competencies, some by the end of the first year of the programme (first 'progression point'), some by the end of second year, others by the end of third year. However, ESCs do not include all the skills and behaviours required of a registered nurse. How competence in ESCs is assessed is discussed in Chapter 6 under assessment of competence.

The competencies under each domain of pre-registration education for midwifery, as well as for SCPHNs, can be viewed in the relevant 'standards of proficiency' or standards documents that are available free from the NMC. 'Standards of proficiency' for the preparation programmes of the AHPs managed by the HPC have also been identified in appropriate HPC publications for each allied health profession that it regulates.

The GMC and General Social Care Council publish similar standards. Other healthcare professions such as clinical perfusion scientists, dance movement therapists, sports therapists and complementary therapists, who normally already have their own separate professional bodies, can join the HPC at some point through a formal application and approval process, and thereafter their standards of proficiencies can be identified. In addition to the regulatory bodies' standards, each healthcare profession's professional body, for example the Royal College of Nursing and the British Medical Association, tend to publish further guidance to facilitate implementation of the regulatory body's standards in professional preparation programmes.

## Why do people learn?

### Activity 2.1    Reasons for learning

Take a step back and consider the learning we undertake in our professional lives, as well as in personal pursuits. Consider examples of what individuals learn, and why. Think of as many reasons as you can for individuals learning various areas of knowledge and skills, and make a list.

It could be argued that everyone learns throughout life – for example, babies learn that when they cry, this leads to food or comfort being made available to them. Younger adults learn new knowledge and skills to enable them, or to improve their chances of, gaining employment and thereby an income to be able to buy food and clothes for themselves, for instance. This could be seen as learning for self-preservation.

Another reason for learning could be self-betterment; self-actualisation is yet another. Professionals might learn more about their profession because they take pride in their craft, and want to acquire comprehensive relevant knowledge. Other reasons for professional and personal learning include:

- Curiosity – about particular subject areas.
- Need for more responsibility – for example, through becoming a practice manager.
- Saving time and effort – students can gain a great deal of knowledge and understanding in one lecture, which would take them a very long time to acquire by self-study.
- Enhancing one's skills – to become even more competent, and even an expert.
- Sense of achievement – for having developed new skills, for instance.
- Acquisition of new skills – in chosen areas of interest.

## The student's learning needs: knowledge and competence

In addition to the placement competencies that students are required to learn, they are likely to have their own aims and thoughts on specific healthcare knowledge and competence that they'd wish to acquire during particular practice placements, as adult learners (Knowles et al., 1998). This should be encouraged and explicitly supported, as appropriate.

Students acquire knowledge in, say, human physiology, pharmacology and treatment methods, which is consistent with the generic and field competencies under the four domains identified by the NMC (2010a). The terms *competence* and *competency* are often used in relation to the skills that students develop. Different types of knowledge are discussed shortly, but first what do the terms 'competence' and 'competency' mean?

### Defining 'competence'
There are conflicting definitions of the terms 'competence' and 'competency' in the literature.

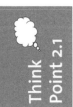

**Think Point 2.1**

## Being competent

Focusing on your own experience of working with colleagues in your healthcare profession, and of students approaching the end of their pre-registration courses, consider what being competent means. For example, which pay band, or what amount of experience makes a healthcare professional 'competent'?

Although the term *competence* is used rather glibly, it is a term that has several definitions, as identified by Bradshaw (1997), for instance. Benner (2001) sees being competent as being at the midway point in the stages of skill acquisition. This is the point when the learner is deemed able to perform the skill safely and effectively unsupervised, but further learning is required to become 'proficient' or 'expert'.

Benner (2001) suggests that competence is an interpretively defined area of skilled performance identified and described by its intent, function and meanings (as in competency statement). Policy and research documents therefore indicate that the terms *competence* and *competent* apply to the person, that is, the professional's overall knowledge, skills and attitudes, and their 'fitness to practise'. The term *competency*, on the other hand, applies to specific clinical skills, which in nursing also include the associated knowledge and attitude components.

The NMC (2005a) identifies competence as relating to the student demonstrating their 'capability' in particular skill areas to a required standard at a particular point in time, and that competencies are component skills that contribute to being competent. A widely accepted definition of competence is 'a term used to describe the skills and ability to practise safely and effectively without the need for direct supervision' (UKCC, 1999: 35). The NMC (2010a: 11) defines it as 'the combination of the skills, knowledge, attitudes, values and technical abilities that underpin safe and effective nursing practice and interventions'. Thus, the concept 'competence' is fundamental to the autonomy and accountability of healthcare professionals, and therefore also to their codes of practice (e.g. NMC, 2008b).

The NMC (2004b) sees a competent nurse as one who consistently demonstrates fitness for practice. Essentially, it can be argued that competence implies being able to perform the clinical intervention safely, confidently and effectively according to the approved procedure or clinical guideline, and without the need for direct supervision. Others argue that competence refers to ability or capability as well as the associated practical knowledge, and yet others feel that competence signifies manifesting theoretical knowledge as well. As a term that is also used in NVQ and in medical education, its profession-specific definition should be accepted, in that in the former the remit for NVQ courses signifies the ability to perform the relevant skill and having the associated practical knowledge. In medical and non-medical professions, competence signifies having the ability, together with the practical and theoretical knowledge.

On the other hand, 'lack of competence' is seen as 'a lack of knowledge, skill or judgement of such a nature that the registrant is unfit to practise safely and effectively in any field in which the registrant claims to be qualified, or seeks practise' (NMC, 2004b: 3). Peers, managers and employers as well as the general public are expected to report lack of competence through the appropriate channels.

## Types of knowledge associated with professional skills

The knowledge required for clinical competence can be grouped or classified in different ways. Schon (1995) notes that healthcare professionals have an accumulated repertoire of knowledge, with mastery over its manipulation, production and application. Benner (2001) identifies practical knowledge and theoretical knowledge, as well as tacit knowledge. She suggests that novices, that is, healthcare professionals who are new to healthcare, are more inclined to use rules and guidelines, such as practical knowledge, while 'expert' healthcare practitioners tend to use intuition more.

Different types of knowledge bases that professionals use can also be viewed from Carper's (1978) 'patterns of knowing' perspective. They are:

- *Empirical knowledge:* knowledge derived from research and scientific experiments, which therefore can be measured, tested and corroborated.
- *Ethical knowledge:* knowledge based on morals and philosophy, but which is usually difficult to test.
- *Aesthetic knowledge:* knowledge based on sensitivity or intuition, such as in the 'art of nursing'.
- *Personal knowledge:* knowledge of one's self and how it influences one's professional practice.

Each of these 'patterns' is seen as equally important for healthcare practice and for developing further knowledge. Therefore in relation to physiotherapy and knowledge regarding hip replacement, for instance, empirical knowledge relates to the research evidence for hip replacement operations, the patient experiencing less chronic pain and a better quality of life afterwards. Ethical knowledge could refer to whether, say, an 80-year-old widow consents to such an operation, and whether it is right to subject her to such a potentially traumatic experience. Aesthetic knowledge refers to the expertise and extensive experience of the physiotherapist to enable the patient to mobilise fully after the operation. Personal knowledge refers to the physiotherapist knowing himself or herself as a person, their preferences and values, and the effect these might have on their professional practice.

The mentor's role towards the physiotherapy student would be to enable the mentee to acquire skills and practical knowledge, but includes having a good insight into the mentee's level of scientific, ethical and personal knowledge.

Alternatively, Scheler (1980) classified knowledge according to the rate at which it alters, that is, according to its 'artificiality'. Technological knowledge such as knowledge of medical devices is seen as the most artificial, as they change frequently through new inventions; knowledge of human anatomy, for instance, is much less artificial.

In a study exploring whether nurses use knowledge from research findings to inform  decision-making, Thompson et al. (2002) found that although colleagues are the more immediate source of information on which to base decisions, they are also a source of research (or data-based empirical) knowledge and useful networks. However, although various decisions made by clinical managers are based on empirical knowledge, other decisions are often influenced by previous experience and intuition.

## Major Views and Perspectives on Learning, Teaching and Education

### What is learning?

How individuals learn has been researched and defined over a number of years. So what is learning? How do you define 'learning'? Generally, dictionaries provide a broad explanation of the term. For instance, to learn is to 'acquire knowledge (of a subject) or skill as a result of study, experience or instruction; to acquire or develop the ability to do' (Brown, 2002: 1562). More specific definitions have come from philosophers and educational psychologists. The latter generally agree that learning is a process that leads to modification in behaviour or the acquisition of new abilities or responses, and which is additional to natural development, growth or maturation.

Accordingly, Gagné (1983) defined learning as a change in human disposition or capability, which persists over a period of time and which is not simply ascribable to the process of growth. Curzon (2003: 12) defines learning as 'the apparent modification of a person's behaviour through his activities and experiences, so that his knowledge, skills and attitudes, including modes of adjustment towards his environment, are changed, more or less permanently'.

These definitions tend to concur that:

- learning is reflected in changes in behaviour, physicality and attitudes;
- learning occurs in day-to-day life experiences, in addition to planned formal education;
- learning a psychomotor skill is permanent in nature in that the individual subsequently has the capacity to perform the skilled act at a future point in time.

Specialist skills may 'decay' mainly due to environmental factors such as changes in medical devices, social values and so on. Learning in healthcare professions is about learning competence and knowledge, the nature of which was discussed earlier. In healthcare professions, learning is a lifelong process of skill and knowledge acquisition and updating them through planned participation in focused reading and structured programmes of study.

## Perspectives on learning

Learning experiences are influenced by where the learner 'is coming from', as each person perceives new experiences in a different way, depending on how they relate to their past. However, two opposing views about formal learning are suggested by Ramsden (2003), who identifies learning as either (a) a quantitative accretion of knowledge, i.e. facts and procedures, or (b) a change in the way in which people interpret and understand the world around them.

Education, on the other hand, according to Socrates (2000 years ago), is not merely transferring knowledge of facts and procedures from 'teacher' to 'pupil'. Rather, it is 'an adventure, an activity of the mind, a pursuit demanding reflection, analysis and investigation, a social activity undertaken by equals freely associated to engage in dialogue' (Jeffs, 2003: 28).

Radical distinctions are also made by Freire (1996), who argues that there are two contrasting perspectives on education and learning, which he identifies as the 'banking' concept of education versus 'problem posing'. The banking concept, as the traditional mode of learning involves the teacher helping a student fill their minds with knowledge, which is later 'cashed out' relatively unchanged, for example in examinations. The problem-posing approach to education, on the other hand, is education through dialogue, in which facilitator and students meet and exchange ideas and experiences through critical discussions and debate. Neither facilitator nor student necessarily has the 'right' answer as there is room for 'multiple realities'.

Another perspective is provided by Peters (1966, 1973) regarding the differentiation between training and education. What distinctions would you draw between education and training? Peters (1966) notes that training means knowledge and skill development devised to bring about some specific end. The aims of education on the other hand, he notes, are that:

- something of value is being passed on and learned;
- the individual comes to care about the learning involved, to develop understanding, and to achieve;
- what is being learned must have a place in a coherent pattern of life, that is, relevance among other things in life.

Therefore, education 'implies that something worthwhile is being, or has been, intentionally transmitted in a morally acceptable manner ... The educated person is one whose life has been transformed by the deepening and widening of his understanding and sensitivity. To be educated is not to arrive at a destination; it is to travel with a different view' (Peters, 1973: 122).

These perspectives on learning correspond with the concepts of teacher-centred learning and student-centred learning, which are discussed in Chapter 3. So how do the definitions and these views on learning and education apply to, or compare with, approaches taken in healthcare profession education curricula?

---

## Activity 2.2   Different perspectives on nurse education

Discuss with a course or work-based peer your thoughts on how far Ramsden's (2003), Freire's (1996) and Peters' (1966, 1973) perspectives on learning apply to nursing, midwifery or to AHP professional education.

---

In nurse education, the difference between education and training is that the word 'training' is usually associated with a well-defined course of action with a definite end point, which is usually that of developing certain pre-defined skills (Burnard and Chapman, 1990). It is said to be a convergent process, in that everyone undertaking the training ends up with mostly the same skills and abilities and the same ways of performing them. Education, on the other hand, is a divergent process of developing and deepening knowledge, skills, interests and values, for instance. Education does not stop at a pre-determined point of attainment, but more in the development of critical ability and, consequently, the individual remains open to new impressions, principles and perspectives. Education facilitators should therefore provide an environment where students feel supported sufficiently to decide on areas and depth of learning, as long as the core curriculum aims are achieved.

## Where do healthcare learners learn?

Naturally, learning doesn't occur only in university classrooms through lectures, workshops and books, but it also occurs in work-based settings, during patient or service user contact. Learning also occurs in skill laboratories and in the ward teaching room or office. Furthermore, learning occurs in the trust's postgraduate or in-service training departments. In the practice setting, learning can take the form of informal and structured teaching sessions.

Furthermore, learning occurs in the student common room, in informal social meetings and even 'in car parks, in corridors, over tea as well as through unnoticed patterns of behaviour and interaction in the classroom itself' (Field, 1999: 12). This notion that learning can occur from friends and peers and in a whole gamut of settings is referred to as social capital (Gopee, 2002a). A corresponding notion is human capital, which refers to self-investment of time and effort by individuals through learning at university or in public libraries, as well as at home, and the non-traditional places suggested by Field (1999). Learning occurs everywhere, including in, for example, therapeutics or propaganda practices. Learning contributes to progress, and notions such as 'learning society' and 'learning organisation' (in that most companies have training and customer services departments) have evolved.

## Theories Underpinning Learning

There are a number of theories of learning that can underpin professional education programmes. Exploration of these theories has taken place over several decades. It has swung between theories of learning, models of learning, principles of learning and styles of learning, with theories and styles of learning being the more popular concepts in the twenty-first century. Further concepts related to learning theories are:

- *Situated learning* – learning in social groups, communal knowledge, apprenticeship.
- *Tacit learning* – knowledge that is implicit and not easily explained.
- *Existential learning* – learning from being and deriving meaning from it.
- *Psychoanalytic learning* – conscious–unconscious dynamics are explored, resulting in a more integrated person.
- *Trait modification* – developing personality characteristics.

The situated learning approach, for instance, comprises learning sub-concepts in social groups or settings, and includes communal knowledge and apprenticeship (Burgoyne and Reynolds, 1997), learning about the ways of the sub-culture, for example in a small community hospital. Other concepts related to learning are: andragogy, student-centred and teacher-centred education, objectives and learning outcomes, taxonomy levels, reflective learning, practice-focused and work-based learning, evidence-based learning, motivation theories and learning by trial and error. Most of these are referred to at appropriate points in the book.

There are at least ten schools of thought, theories or models of learning. They have all created different definitions, and incorporate some of the concepts identified earlier. Most of these theories are developed from the three more robust learning theories, namely:

- behaviourist learning theories;
- cognitive learning theories;
- humanistic learning theories.

## Behaviourist learning theories

Most learning theories belong to the field of psychology, which in the earlier part of the twentieth century used to be about introspection, that is, how mental processes are structured. However, gradually there was a move away from this paradigm (e.g. Watson, 1978) and it was suggested that psychology should be a science, and psychological theories should be based on observable and quantifiable data, that is, those manifested in changes in behaviour. Initially, psychologists worked with animals to observe behaviour changes, and later with people.

Behaviourist learning theories refer to learning through response to particular stimuli, resulting in classical conditioning or operant conditioning. Classical conditioning refers to changes in behaviour through stimulus–response, whereby desirable responses to particular stimuli, that is, newly learned behaviours are rewarded. Operant conditioning is a subsequent development by Skinner (1971) and others, whereby approximations of desired behaviour are rewarded, and thereby the target behaviour develops gradually. Being rewarded for new learning is also known as positive reinforcement, and can be external, in the form of verbal affirmations from the teacher (or close relatives) such as 'well done', or material rewards, or they can be internal through self-satisfaction.

Behaviourist learning theory can be applied to healthcare professionals' education programmes. For instance, operant conditioning can be effectively applied when students with weak academic backgrounds could achieve high levels in academia if earlier attempts are positively reinforced. Overall, healthcare learners are positively reinforced both by feeling a sense of achievement on being able to perform new healthcare skills, and by their mentors/supervisors acknowledging or recognising their newly developed competence.

Another example is that gaining praise for becoming competent at a particular clinical skill, or part-skills towards the desired competent performance, can positively motivate the student and make them want to learn new skills. Thus, praiseworthy performance or approximations of competent practice, or of part-skills, by healthcare learners are rewarded or positively reinforced.

Social learning theory builds on these early behaviourist theories whereby the individual observes competent behaviour or skill performance by professionals, learns and reproduces it, and if the attempt is positively reinforced then that behaviour or skill is likely to be adopted. It refers to behaviour, attitudes and values of teachers or other role models that may be copied by learners (Bandura, 1986, 1997) and thus learned in social situations, as discussed in Chapter 1.

## Cognitive learning theories

As just indicated, behaviourist learning theories initially constituted an attempt to make psychology more scientific and empirical. More recently, various education sectors, including nurse education, have incorporated aspects of behaviourist theories and social learning theory into professional education programmes.

Subsequent work by Piaget (1962), Ausubel et al. (1978) and others led to the evolution of cognitive learning theories, which takes the view that learning is an internal purposive action involving thinking, perception, information processing and memory. Cognitive learning theories include:

- Gestalt theory of learning – entailing insightful learning, the 'aha' phenomenon.
- Ausubel et al.'s (1978) assimilation theory – which incorporates information processing.
- Experiential learning – learning through engaging in practical activities, followed by reflection.

Cognitive learning theories were initially based on animal experiments by Kohler (1925), but all three above-mentioned theories can be applied to healthcare professional education programmes. They include learning by insight (or insightful learning) – gestalt learning theory refers to seeing the whole picture, and insight is gained through the 'aha' phenomenon and the sudden realisation of a solution to a problem, or how various parts fit into a pattern, for instance the 'penny-dropping' experience.

Gestalt theory of learning can be applied to professional education programmes by structuring learning so that learners are given problem situations to resolve, and through group discussions, analysing ideas and trial and error, particular insights are gained. Thus, group discussions, as well as project work, self-directed learning and peer learning can enable this process. Implementation of problem situations that can be used in teaching include, for instance, asking a small group of students to resolve a snapshot of a clinical situation such as helping a patient with partial paralysis move from a bed to a chair.

To a good extent, Bruner's (1960) discovery learning theory refers to insightful learning. It involves situations that are devised in such a way that the learner can discover principles and underlying techniques for themselves. It also involves the use of past experience and existing knowledge to form new insights. For instance, a student who witnesses a patient with asthma gain relief from distressed breathing by using their inhaler can gain further insight into the specific functions of bronchioles and alveoli in oxygen transfer previously encountered in books or lectures.

Ausubel et al.'s (1978) assimilation theory is based on the view that most meaningful cognitive learning takes place as a result of interaction between the knowledge (cognitive structures) the individual already possesses, and new information that the individual encounters. Thus, the single most important factor influencing learning is what the learner already knows. This forms the basis for the transfer of learning, in that, for instance, once the learner comprehends the principles of asepsis in hospital settings, the knowledge can be adapted in community care settings.

Ausubel et al.'s (1978) assimilation theory refers to activating the relevant knowledge the student already has so as to assimilate new knowledge into their existing mental structures. This also increases retention, and is therefore also relevant for adult learners, as they already have substantial knowledge prior to starting on an academic course.

For new information to be 'received and assimilated', or subsumed into an anchoring structure, or schema, Ausubel and colleagues suggest giving the learner prior reading or the opportunity to engage in particular activities in preparation for the teaching session (referred to as 'advanced organisers'). The advanced organiser creates an anchoring structure for the new knowledge, like a scaffolding of ideas on which to build what the student needs to know. For instance, prior to a practice placement with a physiotherapist, the learner could be advised to revise or learn about the microstructure of muscles, in readiness for learning how they are strengthened through exercises by a patient who has had a broken leg operated on.

Cognitive learning theory therefore involves learning by participation and continually taking into consideration the person's previous knowledge and competence, such as clinical skills already learnt by the student on previous placements, and university skills' laboratories.

Experiential learning refers to learning by doing, rather than by merely being informed by others about a particular topic. It is achieved by building simulation activities in teaching–learning sessions, for instance, as advocated by Kolb (1984), among others. Experiential learning is therefore a component of reflective learning.

## Learning from experience

Consider the question 'Do we learn from all experiences we come across in our day-to-day activities?'

Think Point 2.2

In his study of experiences that individuals encounter as they go about their normal day-to-day business, and how much they learn from them, Jarvis (1995) deduced a typology of learning, which identifies three categories and nine types of potential learning experiences as follows:

- *Non-learning*                    Presumption
                                    Non–consideration
                                    Rejection
- *Non-reflective learning*         Preconscious learning
                                    Skills learning
                                    Memorisation
- *Reflective learning*             Contemplation
                                    Reflective skills learning
                                    Experimental learning

The typology also acknowledges the reality that there are particular situations that do not lend themselves to much learning for particular individuals, that is, non-learning experiences. The second category in the typology is non-reflective learning, which includes rote learning and memorising, for example temporary or one-off use of telephone numbers.

However, the third category is reflective learning, which focuses on the important part that experience plays in the learning process. Contemplation refers to thinking about life situations, and hopefully learning from them; and 'experimental learning' refers to learning from findings of well-designed research. Reflective learning refers to the learning that occurs as a result of systematic reflection on situations encountered.

Kolb (1984), for instance, suggests that learning can be conceived as a four-stage learning cycle that involves identifying the immediate concrete experience or an incident as the basis for observation and reflection. Out of this arises new concepts for hypothesis and theory building. Implications of these are considered in new situations and then theory is confirmed, adjusted or advanced.

This form of learning is widely used in general and professional education programmes. Individuals are encouraged to learn from situations or 'critical incidents' they encounter, to analyse them in the context of published literature, and to record them systematically in their portfolios. These can comprise assessed work components of their programme of study.

The rationale for reflective practice in healthcare is that it is also a means of constructing or generating knowledge from particular incidents. The origins of reflection on incidents go back to times when, for instance, techniques for dealing with aggressive behaviour in mental health nursing were minimal. When clinical staff met after such incidents to discuss the situation, they started to realise that if cues and signs of potential violence were identified in the individual patient before the disruptive incident actually occurred, then they could take certain actions to prevent it happening in the first place. This was formalized and seen as a therapeutic means that could be used, step-by-step, to prevent the disruptive incident. This also constituted constructing knowledge from clinical practice. The lack of knowledge and theory development from day-to-day experiences in practice settings was a weakness identified by Phillips et al.'s (2000) study of mentoring practices.

Similar 'concrete experiences' led to changes in clinical practice such as use of the triage system in Accident and Emergency departments, ensuring normal saline solution is at room temperature or above, prior to using it for wound cleansing. Several of these examples are noted in Chapter 5.

Kolb's (1984) learning cycle comprises four stages in the learning process, from the initial concrete experience or incident, through to retrospectively exploring the experience so that it leads to new learning, generalising from the new learning, to applying new learning to similar new situations. The original Kolbs' cycle is presented as a closed circle with the fourth stage (applying new learning) leading to the first (the initial concrete experience). However, it is likely that the new learning may not be fully effective when applied to new situations that are similar, or even identical, to the initial concrete experience or incident, and therefore it becomes another new experience or incident to learn from. Consequently, the experiential learning cycle can be presented more meaningfully as a spiral that shows that applying new learning to similar situations must be undertaken with an open mind, as further learning might ensue in the light of new evidence and evolving social changes, as well as possibly research (see Figure 2.1).

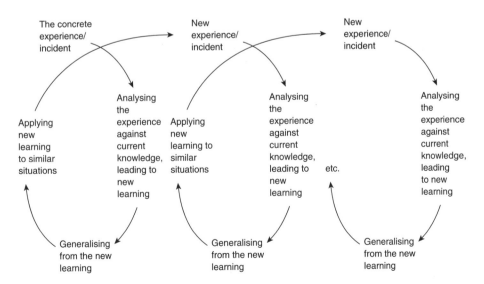

FIGURE 2.1   The experiential learning spiral

Adapting (i.e. making small changes) to published models and frameworks in one's teaching and learning is not uncommon, and can in fact be recommended as they are applied to specific groups of people or activities. This is also because Kolb's model of learning has its critics. For example, Bergsteiner et al. (2010) thoroughly examined Kolb's learning cycle, and argue that the graphics of the model are flawed, and suggest changes. Rogers and Horrocks (2010) argue that since learning from new experiences requires 'critical reflection', all learning cycles need to be adapted in the search for new principles before new conclusions are reached.

Nonetheless, teachers and students can alternatively utilise other models of reflection, such as one by Boud et al. (1985), Gibbs (1988), or others that are generally available in the literature. Boud and colleagues' model of reflective practice involves identifying the concrete experience, observation and reflections, attending to feelings, re-evaluating the experience and new learning.

For instance, when the student encounters a new experience during the practice placement, they observe the experience as a critical incident and later they recall the incident, and describe it, reflect on it and explore it in the context of existing knowledge within professional and other relevant literature. As a result of this, they develop and generate further insight by identifying and redefining the problem in a climate of mutual support (at university reflection-on-action workshops, for instance). They can share their new-found knowledge in as much detail as appropriate, even make a presentation, as it might have teaching implications for future practice. However, to benefit from this concept, the scheduling of the learning process should ensure that time is made available following practice placements for reflection, consolidation and evaluation.

### Constructivism

Also gaining in popularity is a further development from the three groups of cognitive learning theories, which is known as 'constructivism'. As a concept that was earlier pioneered by Berger and Luckmann (1967) as the social construction of reality, constructivism earlier signified how individuals construct new thoughts, images, concepts and theories, that is 'scaffolded' onto the individual's existing current and past knowledge. Such knowledge is based on both social experiences and encounters with learning.

Currently, as a learning theory, constructivism is founded on the premise that, by reflecting on our experiences, we construct our own unique understanding of learning encounters, and in the quest for meaning we construct our own images and models of reality. Thereby the student does not accept verbatim all knowledge presented to them, but assimilates them in the context of their prior knowledge.

## Humanistic learning theories

A third group of theories that have been developed with regards to how learning occurs is humanistic learning theories, which include:

- Alan Rogers' characteristics of adult education and andragogy;
- Carl Rogers' student-centred approach to learning;
- Maslow's learning as self-actualisation.

Humanistic learning theorists claim that preceding theories omit aspects of human existence such as feelings, attitudes and values, and thereby overlook the more holistic perspective that incorporates attitudinal components of learning. They suggest that learning should be concerned with personal human growth. Students can therefore learn concepts, theories, models and propositions (i.e. 'propositional knowledge') from books and other learning resources, and spend more classroom time on experiential learning activities, which include thinking processes that also incorporate exploration of values, attitudes and feelings.

### Adults as students

In the context of the more holistic and humanistic approaches to learning, adult learning is another concept in its own right.

## Adult learners

Consider the question 'Should ways of teaching adults be different from ways of teaching school children or college students?'. That is, what is different about adult students in contrast to school or college pupils? Think of reasons for your answer.

**Think Point 2.3**

Rogers and Horrocks (2010), Mezirow (1983) and Knowles et al. (1998) suggest various ways in which teaching adults, or adult education, is different from teaching children. Teaching adults includes teaching university students on generic or professional courses. Some of the differences suggested by nurses on post-registration courses are identified in Table 2.1.

However, in both instances, the learner–teacher relationship is important and needs to be based on mutual trust. Different teachers may have their own repertoire of different teaching styles and techniques when teaching adult students. Rogers and Horrocks (2010) conclude by identifying the characteristics of adult students or learners, as individuals who:

**TABLE 2.1**   Differences in ways in which adults and children learn

| How children learn | How adults learn |
| --- | --- |
| Children have shorter attention span, and therefore a variety of learning activities is needed, including starter activities. | Adults are (usually) self-motivated to learn. |
| | Adults may have relevant (or faulty) professional and life experiences. |
| Teaching children is pedagogy, e.g. telling them. | Open discussion is more feasible in adult groups. |
| Children are more open to new ideas. | Lesson content can be adjusted based on ongoing evaluation of learning needs. |
| There is a need to reinforce information over time. | |

*Source*: Gopee, 2000

- define themselves, and have a self-image as adult students;
- are in the middle of a process of growth, not at the start of the process;
- bring with them a package of experience and values;
- come to learning with intentions;
- bring with them expectations about the learning process;
- have competing interests;
- already have their own set of patterns of learning.

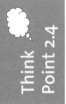

**Think Point 2.4**

## Adult education in healthcare courses

How far is the adult learning approach relevant or applicable to nursing and other AHP education?

Adult education is defined by Mezirow (1983) as an organised and sustained effort to assist adults to learn in a way that enhances their capacity to function as self-directed learners. Both Mezirow's definition and Rogers and Horrocks' characteristics of adult learners suggest that adult students' learning can be facilitated more effectively within an ethos of self-directed learning. Mentors can build self-directed learning into practice placement programmes for learners by allocating time for exploring further relevant clinical experiences or consulting relevant learning resources.

### Andragogy and self-directed learning

Andragogy is an approach to teaching and learning aimed at enabling individuals to become aware that they should be the originators of their own thinking. Accordingly, although substantial knowledge and skill acquisition begins on qualifying (e.g. becoming a registered nurse), it is up to the individual professional to determine the necessary areas of learning for themselves.

This learning could be instigated by ward-based experiences, and the self-direction developed should become career-long.

In a qualitative study of lecturers' and students' perceptions of self-directed learning and factors that facilitate or impede them, Lunyk-Child et al. (2001) found that students who engage in self-directed learning undergo a transformation that begins with negative feelings (i.e. confusion, frustration and dissatisfaction), but ends with confidence and skills for lifelong learning.

However, another side to self-directed learning is highlighted by Hughes (1999) who indicates that this approach is not necessarily 'emancipatory', as it can be a 'repressive instrument' in that it can marginalise the importance of collective and co-operative learning, that is, learning in groups in classrooms. Hughes suggests that governments can use self-directed learning to argue that less central funding would be required to educate self-directed learners. Furthermore, Knowles et al. (1998) suggest that the teacher needs to develop specific competencies to implement self-directed learning effectively. In the light of these issues and reservations related to andragogy, and the benefits, and Rogers and Horrocks' (2010) general characteristics of adult learners, it can be concluded that in healthcare:

- Adult education constitutes collaborative activities by teachers and learners.
- Teaching should build on learners' professional experiences.
- Learners should participate in identifying learning needs, setting objectives and evaluating learning.
- The level of effective application of theory to clinical practice must always be identified.
- The role of the teacher is that of a facilitator.
- The outcome of the teaching and learning encounter should be to enable the individual to develop into a responsible autonomous practitioner.

## Student-centred teaching

Carl Rogers (1983) is well known for suggesting that teaching may be an overrated activity, as it is learning that should be in focus. For this to happen, he advocated the use of empathic understanding, genuineness and being non-judgemental in learning situations. These activities are helping skills that Rogers successfully transferred from therapeutic counselling situations to student-learning situations (Rogers and Freiberg, 1994). The teacher thus becomes the facilitator of student-centred learning, as is also advocated by Knowles et al. (1998) and Freire (1996). The facilitator achieves this by creating the environment for learning and identifying resources, and therefore empowering students to become responsible, to develop self-awareness and to think of alternatives. Student-centred teaching is discussed in some detail in Chapter 3.

## Learning and self-actualisation

Maslow's (1987) theory of a hierarchy of human needs suggests that our highest-level need, which is also lower priority, is our need for self-actualisation. Our physiological needs are highest priority, followed by safety needs, the need for belongingness and love, our self-esteem needs, and finally the need for self-actualisation. It could be argued that the goal of education is to assist individuals to achieve self-actualisation, to help the person to become the best that they are able to become with the resources that are accessible. Maslow observed that the characteristics of self-actualising individuals are that they:

- have a more efficient perception of reality;
- demonstrate acceptance of self and others;
- show spontaneity, simplicity and naturalness;
- are problem-centred;
- possess a quality of detachment and have a need for privacy;
- exercise autonomy, independence of culture and environment;
- show continued freshness of appreciation;
- have peak experiences;
- experience deeper, more profound interpersonal relations;
- demonstrate democratic character;
- have a philosophical, non-hostile sense of humour;
- show creativeness;
- seem to transcend any culture.

Teachers might argue that they apply the above-mentioned theories of learning as appropriate, with particular groups or with individual learners. However, from adult educators' professional perspectives, andragogy also requires consideration of whether the adult student is merely biologically adult, or merely of legally adult age, or is also being a psychologically and socially responsible adult.

Furthermore, Race (2010: viii) reviewed the main prevailing theories of learning, and observed that most theories are worded in academic technical language used by educational psychologists that the majority of readers find cumbersome, and not easy to comprehend. He therefore constituted his theory of learning using much simpler words, which he termed 'ripples on a pond' model of learning, which in turn identifies fundamental factors underpinning successful learning, namely:

- wanting to learn;
- taking ownership of the need to learn;
- learning by doing;
- learning through feedback;

- making sense of what is being learned;
- explaining, or teaching or coaching;
- making informed judgements – assessing.

The ripples model of learning is a more recent further development of experiential learning, and is therefore rooted in 'learning by doing'. Race argues that the seven factors underpinning learning occur in sequence, with each stage interacting with those next to it, much like a pebble falling into a pond and creating ripples with each stage moving in backward and forward directions. It is presented as concentric circles. It is interesting to note that the first three 'ripples' tend to represent learners' motivation and the actions that they take to learn, both being components that have featured for decades as crucial for effective learning.

Race's ripples model of learning can be implemented in educating healthcare profession students by ensuring that each factor is achieved, such as enabling students to become motivated to learn, creating the medium for 'learning by doing' by giving feedback, and creating opportunities for students to teach others.

## How Else do We Learn Healthcare Skills?

In addition to different theories of learning, learning is also influenced by the different styles and approaches to learning adopted by individuals. The distinctions between theories and styles can be explained as follows.

A theory tends to imply cause and effect, that is, if we do x, then y will happen. For instance, if the Smiths send their child to an independent school, then he/she will have a better chance of securing a student place in a reputable university. According to the dictionary (Brown, 2002: 3236) a theory is 'a systematic statement of rules or principles to be followed; a system of ideas or statement explaining something, especially one based on general principles, independent of the thing to be explained'. Alternatively, Lindberg et al. (1998: 62) define a theory as 'a group of concepts, definitions, and statements that presents an organised view of phenomena ... with the intent of describing, explaining, or controlling these phenomena'. A learning theory, the humanistic theory for instance, comprises an organised view of a group of concepts that should result in much more effective learning.

In contrast to a learning theory, a learning style refers to the unique way in which the particular individual tends to respond to learning situations so that they acquire the targeted skill or knowledge. For instance, do they accept new learning instantly, or do they prefer to reflect on it before accepting it fully? Do they question first whether the learning has practical applications or do they accept new concepts at theoretical levels first? Alternatively, approaches to learning tend to depend on the level of individual commitment to particular episodes of learning, as discussed shortly in this chapter.

## Major learning styles

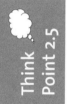

**Think Point 2.5**

## How do you prefer to learn? What is your learning style?

We are all unique as learners. How does each of us prefer to learn? What is your preferred learning style? Which style does not suit you?

Learning styles have been researched over a number of years, and Honey and Mumford's (2000) classification of styles of learning is one that has been most widely published. You might have responded to Think Point 2.5 by identifying that you prefer to learn by attending a course or lecture, that is, in formal teaching situations. Others may prefer to learn by:

- watching others, and seeing the end-product first;
- trial and error, generally through experience;
- reading, and other forms of personal study such as distance learning;
- discussion with others.

Another well accepted proponent of learning styles is Kolb (1984), whose theory of learning and identification of learning styles is based on a view of learning as a series of experiences with cognitive additions to existing psychological structures. There are some similarities in the way Kolb and then Honey and Mumford group different learning styles. Kolb suggests that there are four styles of learning manifested by students, namely the converger, the diverger, the assimilator and the accommodator. Honey and Mumford (2000) suggest that individual learners vary between whether they are activists, reflectors, theorists or pragmatists. Jarvis and Gibson (1997) add other learning styles such as focusers, scanners, impulsivity and reflectivity. The main learning styles are summarised in Box 2.2.

---

## Box 2.2   Major learning styles

| | |
|---|---|
| Converger vs Diverger | Convergers are individuals who tend to use abstract thinking, progress to active experimentation, and generate a single correct solution; divergers tend to start from concrete experiences, generate ideas, then speculate on broader perspectives. |
| Impulsivity vs Reflectivity (similar to Accommodator vs Assimilator) | Using the 'impulsive' style means the individual tends to respond first, at times spontaneously, and reflect later; those who use reflectivity tend to reflect first and respond subsequently. |
| Activists vs Reflectors | Individuals who are activitists tend to involve themselves fully in new experiences; reflectors ponder on experiences from different perspectives, thoroughly analysing them, before participating in the experience in practice. |
| Theorists vs Pragmatists | Theorists are individuals who start from observations, and develop or synthesise them into theories; pragmatists tend to consider the practical application of novel encounters first, and theorise afterwards. |
| Focuser vs Scanner | Focusers are individuals who examine the whole problem and develop solutions from them; scanners tend to solve one aspect of the problem at a time, and assume it is the correct one unless it is disproved. |
| Holistic vs Serialistic | Individuals using the holistic approach tend to prefer to see a phenomenon as a whole, while serialists prefer to identify its components and their roles as part of the whole phenomenon. |

---

Styles of learning are explained in full detail in relevant literature. For instance, the style *Impulsivity vs Reflectivity* implies that some individuals respond to new learning stimuli first and reflect later, while other individuals reflect first and respond afterwards. Although the latter might be intellectually sounder, the former has its uses in certain situations, especially by those who are in a position to use intuitive knowledge.

To enable utilisation of styles of learning, Honey and Mumford (2000) designed a Learning Style Questionnaire (LSQ) which is widely used. The LSQ constitutes a self-assessment tool that indicates which style is generally utilised by the individual completing it, and the main uses of knowledge derived from the LSQ are:

- Increased awareness of learning activities that are congruent with the individual's learning style.
- A better choice of activities leading to more effective and economical learning.
- Identification of areas in which an individual's less effective learning processes can be improved.
- Development of ways in which specific learning skills can be improved, for example reflective learning.

A number of questionnaires and inventories on learning styles are available in education literature and through the internet, but research on learning styles almost always indicate that students do not choose and use only one style of learning, as they use different ones, or a combination of styles. James et al. (2011), for instance, explored the learning styles of first-year nursing and midwifery students utilising the VARK (visual, aural, read–write and kinaes-thetic) questionnaire, and found that the majority of students were 'multi-modal', that is they use all four modes of learning identified in VARK. Fleming et al.'s (2011) longitudinal study also concluded that student nurses do not use one 'dominant learning style' although they do recognise that educators should be aware of students' learning styles, and endeavour to maximise students' learning potential by utilising a range of teaching and learning methods.

### Adapting to students' styles of learning

Despite research findings, it is arguable that, where feasible, the mentor should endeavour to be aware of their mentee's learning style and approach to see if they can adapt to them to make their teaching more effective. This could make the achievement of practice objectives easier and more efficient.

An example of the adaptation of the *Theorists vs Pragmatists* style of learning is as follows. For instance, if the mentor finds that a particular student has leanings towards the pragmatist style, for any particular component of learn-ing, that is, they immediately want to know how the learning applies to actual patient or service user care situations, then the mentor can focus on the practical application of the learning first, moving on to underpinning theo-ries afterwards. The practical knowledge can follow immediately afterwards, and the theoretical knowledge later. Another student may wish to acquire all necessary theoretical knowledge before engaging in its practical application.

However, individual learning styles are not fixed, as the individual may consciously change their learning style according to the situation. Learners could, as noted above, develop their ability in all styles of learning, and change or adapt them as new knowledge and skills are encountered, which might depend on how novel the new experience is to the individual. Style may also change through new experiences and at different stages of maturation.

## Students with special educational needs

In addition to theories and individual styles of learning, facilitators of learning should also heed the special education needs (SEN) of individual students. The number of students disclosing that they have a disability is increasing, including those who are students on healthcare profession courses. Universities have an obligation to comply with legal requirements, such as those of the Disability Discrimination Act (DDA) (Office of Public Sector Information (OPSI), 2005), and the Special Education Needs and Disability Act (OPSI, 2001), which are now incorporated in the Equality Act 2010 (Equality Challenge Unit, 2010). As it is mandatory for students to acquire professional skills in practice settings for a specified number of hours during the course (e.g. NMC, 2010a), mentors have to be aware of their obligations towards students with disabilities as well under these Acts.

The QAA (2010: 7) prefers to refer to the student with SENs as 'disabled student' but retains the DDA's (OPSI, 2005) definition of disability. The Equality Act defines disability very similarly as 'a physical or mental impairment, which has a substantial and long term adverse effect on his or her ability to carry out normal day to day activities'.

The above-mentioned Acts also identify a list of different impairments that constitute a disability, including dyslexia, visual or hearing impairment, mental health conditions, etc. In addition to disabilities, the Equality Act, which came into force on 1 October 2010, encompasses other human characteristics that employers could willingly or inadvertently discriminate against. It identifies nine such 'protected characteristics', namely:

- Age
- Disability
- Gender assignment
- Marriage and civil partnership
- Pregnancy and maternity
- Race
- Religion or belief (including lack of belief)
- Sex
- Sexual orientation

Furthermore, the above Acts indicate that institutions must make 'reasonable adjustments' to support students with SENs' learning and assessment. Almost all organisations concerned with education of healthcare profession students make their own written statement on how they make 'reasonable adjustments', including the RCN (2007) and the QAA (2010). The RCN's guidance on how reasonable adjustments can be made in the practice setting for students with dyslexia is as follows (2007: 19–20):

- the use of coloured overlays to assist in reading text on white paper
- the use of coloured paper
- additional training and support
- giving verbal rather than written instructions
- allowing plenty of time to read and complete the task
- giving instructions one at a time, slowly and clearly, in a quiet location
- reminding the person of important deadlines and reviewing priorities regularly
- using a wall planner, and creating a 'to do' list
- the use of modified/specialised equipment
- provision of a quiet area to write up notes, or for when specific tasks require intense concentration
- flexible working hours/frequent breaks.

For advice and support on how to make adjustments for students with SEN, mentors can consult various named individuals and departments such as the local university's lecturer(s) who specialises in this topic area, Occupational Health services, students' unions, etc.

Research on the extent to which the needs of students with SENs are met include those by White (2007) and Tee et al. (2010). White, for instance, conducted a qualitative study to explore how far the education needs of students with dyslexia are met during their pre-qualifying programme. She found that students experienced particular problems during practice placements, but none of the mentors in the study felt adequately educationally prepared to help students with disabilities. Students with SENs do develop their own coping strategies, and the study recommends that more concerted effort should be made to support both students and their mentors to make the necessary 'reasonable adjustments'.

Griffiths et al. (2010) provide a six-phase framework for supporting disabled students systematically for more effective learning during practice placements. However, other than in the context of policies related to disabilities, there is also an abundance of literature and research on the topic area. Scullion (2010), for instance, identifies the two most prominent perspectives on disability, the medical model and the social model. As the term implies, the medical model endeavours to enable people with disabilities to function to their maximum by rectifying the problem as far as they can at the patho-physiological level. The social model tends to view those with disabilities as ones who should not be stereotyped and stigmatised, but adjustments made to their social environment to enable them to function to their maximum. Scullion indicates that, as a strategy to challenge discrimination, healthcare professionals should promote and enhance the social model of disability through 'social advocacy'.

However, a literature review of 'reasonable adjustments in nursing and midwifery' conducted on behalf of the NMC by Kane and Gooding (2009: 19–21) revealed that there are still various issues related to this, including the resources required for reasonable adjustments to be made, non-disclosure of a disability for fear of social discrimination, etc. Furthermore, as Tee et al. (2010) found that disabled students require 20 per cent more contact time with lecturers than non-disabled peers, they recommend the appointment of a 'student practice learning advisor' whose primary role will be to support disabled students by ensuring opportunities to succeed are maximised by operationalising recommended adjustments in practice.

## Approaches to learning

Evolving from different theories and styles, research has also identified different approaches to learning. Marton et al.'s (1997) research on approaches to learning identified individuals who take a deep approach to learning, those who take a surface approach and those who take the strategic approach. Students tend to use one of these three approaches. The defining features of each approach are presented in Box 2.3.

---

**Box 2.3   Deep, surface and strategic approaches to learning**

| Deep approach | Relates ideas to previous knowledge and experience |
| --- | --- |
| | Looks for patterns and underlying principles |
| | Checks evidence and relates it to conclusions |
| | Examines logic and argument cautiously and critically |
| | Engages with full interest with the course content |
| Surface approach | Studies without reflecting on purpose and strategy |
| | Treats the course as unrelated bits of knowledge (discrete elements) |
| | Memorises facts and procedures in relation to assessments |
| | Finds difficulty in making sense of new ideas presented |
| | Feels undue pressure and worry about coursework |

*(Continued)*

---

*(Continued)*

| Strategic approach | Puts consistent effort into studying |
|---|---|
| | Ensures conditions and materials for studying are appropriate |
| | Manages or organises time and effort to greatest effect |
| | Is alert to assessment requirements and criteria, and pays attention to cues about marking schemes |
| | Gears work to the perceived preferences of lecturers |

---

Whether a student takes the deep or surface approach to learning (Marton et al., 1997) might also depend on the stage of development of the subject area. Social sciences and arts may warrant a deep approach, while parts of science subjects such as biology and law might only require surface approaches, at least at earlier stages because they often constitute factual, single-answer knowledge. Newer and less factual subjects might also warrant a deep approach.

Approaches to learning also relate to the quality of the learning undertaken. Ramsden (2003) reports that if someone treated learning as an external imposition and concentrated on memorising facts, then that person was taking a surface approach to learning, and this would result in poor knowledge and understanding of the subject. Alternatively, 'if they intended to understand and interacted vigorously with the content of the text (a deep approach), they stood a better chance of getting the author's message and being able to remember the supporting facts' (2003: 19). As for adapting to the student's approach to learning, the mentor would prefer the student to take a deep approach but, during very busy times, strategic and surface approaches might temporarily be relevant.

## Principles of learning

Based on the views, theories, styles and approaches to learning discussed in this chapter, there are certain generally agreed principles of learning that can be concluded from them, which can make learning more effective, from both facilitators' and learners' standpoints. Mostly derived from Gagné (1983) and Knowles et al. (1998), these are:

- Whatever a student learns, they must actively learn it themselves – no one can learn it for them.
- Each student learns at their own chosen pace, as this varies depending on their particular circumstances, mental abilities and various other factors.

- A student learns more when each step is immediately reinforced or corrected.
- Full, rather than partial, mastery of each step makes the total more meaningful.
- When given responsibility for their own learning, the student can become more highly motivated and likely to learn and retain more.
- The teacher as manager of learning should assume that McGregor's (1987) theory Y prevails, that is, learners are self-motivated to learn, and they seek out learning opportunities for themselves (theory X implies learners have to be directed or coerced to learn).
- Students who come to education expecting to be passively fed information and knowledge should be eased into andragogical principles of learning and teaching soon after.

## Chapter Summary

This chapter has focused predominantly on the what and how of learning professional knowledge and competence, and has therefore explored:

- What healthcare learners learn, and why, in the context of the student's learning needs in relation to knowledge and competence, and the different types of knowledge associated with professional skills.
- The definitions of competence and healthcare competencies, and issues related to them.
- Major views and perspectives on learning, teaching and education, which include what learning is, and where and how individual healthcare learners learn.
- Theories underpinning learning, in particular behaviourist learning theories (including Bandura's social learning theory), cognitive learning theories, and humanistic learning theories such as andragogy and self-directed learning, student-centred approach to learning, and learning as self-actualisation.
- How learners learn healthcare skills, which included an examination of major styles of learning, and approaches to learning, such as deep, surface and strategic learning, and how the mentor could adapt their mentoring activities to students' individual styles and approaches; and strategies for facilitating learning for students with SEN.

## Further Optional Reading

For full details of all the NMC's requirements for effective and quality-assured pre-registration nurse education in the UK, see:

- Nursing and Midwifery Council (2010a) *Standards for Pre-registration Nursing Education*. Available at: http://standards.nmc-uk.org/PreRegNursing/Pages/Introduction.aspx. Accessed 18 September 2010.

For a detailed discussion on 'vicarious learning' in relation to social learning theory, see:

- Bandura, A. (1997) *Self-Efficacy – The Exercise of Control*. New York: W H Freeman and Company, pp. 86–101.

- Roberts, D. (2010) 'Vicarious learning: A review of the literature', *Nurse Education in Practice*, 10 (1): 13–16.

For optional activity, in the context of Kolb's experiential learning cycle, think of two activities in practice settings in which previous learning from similar incidents or situations did not apply fully to subsequent situations, and what action was, or could have been, taken as a result of this.

For career progression of students with special education needs, see also:

- Morris, D. and Turnbull, P. (2007) 'A survey based exploration of the impact of dyslexia on the career progression of registered nurses in the UK', *Journal of Nursing Management*, 15 (1): 97–106.

For updates on the current provision for students with SEN, and detailed guidance on how to support learning for students with disabilities, see:

- Quality Assurance Agency for Higher Education (2010) *Code of Practice for the Assurance of Academic Quality and Standards in Higher Education Section 3: Disabled students*. Available at: www.qaa.ac.uk/academicinfrastructure/codeofpractice/section3/section3disabilities2010.pdf. Accessed 3 July 2010.

Learning styles' questionnaires and inventories are easily accessible on the internet through one of the search engines such as Google. See also the following research article on the VARK learning styles:

- James, S., D'Amore, A. and Thomas, T. (2011) 'Learning preferences of first year nursing and midwifery students: Utilising VARK', *Nurse Education Today*.

# 3
# Facilitating Learning

## Introduction

Having explored in Chapter 1 what mentoring, preceptoring and similar roles signify, the reasons for the mentor role and how it can be performed effectively, and then in Chapter 2 the different major perspectives on learning, along with learning theories, styles and approaches, this chapter focuses on the teaching and facilitation of learning roles of the mentor. Over the years, both the UKCC and the NMC have implicated the mentor as the main 'teacher' in practice settings. This chapter therefore considers the various professional groups of learners whose learning healthcare professionals facilitate; whether to teach or facilitate learning; systematic ways of facilitating learners' acquisition of practice skills and knowledge; as well as some of the main issues related to facilitation of learning in practice settings. The mentor's competence under the 'facilitation of learning' domain and the related outcomes identified by the NMC (2008a) were noted in the introduction section of Chapter 2.

## Chapter outcomes

On completion of this chapter, you should be able to:

1  Identify a wide range of students and learners whose learning qualified healthcare professionals facilitate.
2  Differentiate between teaching and facilitation of learning, as well as different perceptions of teaching, taking into account prominent contemporary approaches to teaching and learning.
3  Evaluate a number of ways in which mentors can enable healthcare profession students and learners to acquire health and social care skills, the steps involved in effective planning for skills teaching, along with the underpinning knowledge base.

4   Ascertain structured and systematic methods of teaching that can be implemented by
    mentors to enable students and learners to acquire health profession skills and knowledge.
5   Evaluate various methods of teaching and presentation aids that can be selected for
    effective teaching, and also ways of managing some of the likely problems with them.

## Whose Learning do Healthcare Professionals Facilitate, and Why?

---

### Activity 3.1    Whom do healthcare professionals teach?

To start exploring facilitation of learning, first make a list of all groups of
people whom nurses and other healthcare professionals teach. Having
done this, add the exact healthcare topic areas that they are likely to teach
to the different groups of individuals.

---

The healthcare professional's role includes a substantial teaching component,
and therefore you might have felt that Activity 3.1 was rather simplistic. It
does reflect, however, the reality of the extent of teaching that RNs and RMs
do, and in response to the activity, you might have mentioned:

* Nurses teaching student nurses (first, second and third year), healthcare assistants on
  national vocational qualification courses, patients/service users, patient's relatives, and
  junior doctors.
* Midwives teach women/service users, for example new mothers and fathers, how to
  look after a new baby.
* The practice nurse teaches primary (and secondary) level ill-health prevention, for
  example how to quit smoking, lose weight, expectant mothers regarding their diet,
  and relaxation for those with high blood pressure.
* SCPHNs teach mothers with different needs, such as single teenage mothers or those
  in different age groups.

## Why do healthcare professionals need to know how to facilitate learning?

On a day-to-day basis, the healthcare professional's role focuses largely on
attending to patients' and service users' health problems. Teaching activities
generally tend to be more transient, and are engaged in at opportune moments.

Nevertheless, there are several reasons why healthcare professionals teach and facilitate learning. First, in addition to teaching colleagues and juniors being a job requirement for most healthcare professionals by virtue of their contract of employment, it also constitutes one of the four essential components of nursing and midwifery, as identified by Wright (1990), the Scottish Government (2010) and in DH policy documents, the other components being clinical practice, care organisation and involvement in research. Correspondingly, the *NHS KSF* (DH, 2004a: 57) notes under 'personal and people development' that healthcare professionals have to contribute to 'the development of others during ongoing work activities [by] structured approaches … informal and ad hoc methods …', and demonstrate and share skills and knowledge.

Similarly, teaching usually forms part of healthcare professionals' codes of practice, which stipulate that they must be willing to share skills and experience. For instance, the NMC's (2008b: 5) code of practice specifies that the RN 'must be willing to share [your] skills and experience for the benefit of your colleagues', and has 'a duty to facilitate students and others to develop their competence'. This form of teaching includes teaching new skills to colleagues (RNs/RMs), for example the use of new medical devices such as a new glucometer, how to conduct a patient assessment, the Doppler technique; and teaching healthcare profession students.

Teaching is also an integral component of healthcare professionals' pre-registration education programmes as identified by the NMC (2010a), under the domain 'Communication and interpersonal skills', for instance, indicating that nurses must educate patients and service users 'to encourage health promoting behaviour' (2010a:16); and under 'Leadership, management and team-working', 'All nurses must facilitate nursing students and others to develop their competence using a range of professional and personal development skills' (2010a: 20).

Furthermore, specialist RNs and other healthcare professionals are at times required, or invited, to do small-group teaching on specific aspects of their specialist areas, within the healthcare trust, or classroom teaching on specialist university-based courses.

Additionally, healthcare professionals might also engage in teaching merely to advance the teaching or presentation skills that they have previously acquired to varying degrees. They could thereby also start to develop public-speaking skills. For more experienced mentors, teaching provides them with an opportunity to apply the principles of teaching and learning, and experiment with new teaching techniques. Furthermore, mentors have to teach because of variable levels of success in joint education-trust roles such as lecturer–practitioners and the clinical teaching role of nurse lecturers.

## Facilitating Learning or Teaching?

At times, we hear the statement, 'John (or Jane) is an excellent (or a born) teacher,' but, as with most skills, teaching can be regarded as an 'art' and a 'science'. This means that although someone may appear to have a natural knack for teaching, it is also a skill that can be learned, using scientifically deduced theories. Short or long teaching courses such as the City and Guilds 7307 *Certificate in Teaching Adult Learners*, and the *Post-graduate Certificate in Education* courses, are designed specifically for this purpose. After several years of teaching experience, eventually the skill becomes so well developed and refined that it appears akin to an artistic talent. However, thinking about some of the concepts discussed in Chapter 2, such as self-directed learning and reflective learning, consider the question 'Should mentors teach mentees and juniors, or facilitate their learning?' Both concepts are suggested for contemporary mentoring activities.

## Approaches to teaching and learning

Dictionaries tend to define teaching as 'to tell or show, to give instruction or lessons in' or 'to enable (a person) to do something by instruction and training'. Such definitions tend to signify teaching as one-way traffic, that is, the teacher controls the content, direction and flow of the session's content. It also reflects one of the earlier approaches to teaching. However, various other approaches to teaching and learning have evolved over the years, so much so that Joyce et al. (2009) indicate that there are more than 22 models of teaching, some of which are well researched, whilst others still need rigorous testing.

An underlying trend that figures clearly in all these approaches and models of teaching, is the transition from the rather derogatory term 'teacher-centred' teaching to 'student-centred' teaching. Three stages of evolution of approaches to teaching can be identified, which are as follows.

1   In the earlier stage, teaching was seen as the teacher imparting selected and predetermined knowledge and skills to students as he or she is the expert in that subject area. In such approaches, students in turn are passive recipients of the instruction, but this results in students feeling inhibited from exploring alternative views.

2   In a gradual change in attitude towards teaching and learning, teaching was viewed as enabling active learning, an approach in which teachers structure learning activities for students so that the latter actively engage with the subject matter and explore specific topic areas in the curriculum or syllabus. Thus, the teacher leads students to conclusions by enquiry and questioning.

3   In the third and current stage, teaching is viewed as 'facilitating learning', whereby teachers work in partnership with students and jointly determine their learning needs

in the overall context of the curriculum, and the means by which those learning needs will be met. The teacher creates the conditions for learning and does not control all learning outcomes, thus allowing the student a substantial degree of choice in what to learn.

These three stages of development in ways of teaching therefore reflect an evolving trend from the earlier one implying a teacher-centred approach, to the latter being much more student centred, and therefore progressing from teaching to facilitation of learning. The approach chosen of course depends on several factors such as the particular student group's motivation to learn, the teacher's own beliefs about teaching and learning, and the subject matter, or a deliberate combination of these as the teacher feels appropriate.

The three teaching approaches can also be categorised as didactic, Socratic or facilitative, respectively. Contemporarily, Ramsden (2003) refers to these approaches as theories 1, 2 and 3, whilst Biggs and Tang (2007: 15–19) interpret these three approaches to three 'levels of thinking about teaching', and note that in stage (or level) one, if the student does not 'absorb' the knowledge and skills imparted to the student, either because they haven't got the ability or the motivation to do so, then the teaching is unlikely to be effective.

In the level (or stage) two approach, in addition to the ability to impart knowledge and skills, the teacher needs additional skills such as the ability to structure learning activities and to negotiate student learning so as to ensure the curriculum's learning outcomes are met. Yet further skills are required in the third and current level of thinking about teaching, which is facilitation of learning as this is based on the student's own learning needs, and is about enabling students to engage with their learning more actively. The earlier approaches were also reflected in the method of assessment used by educators, which had negative effects on students' learning and achievement.

The trend in moving away from teacher-centred approaches to student-centred ones was suggested several years ago by Bruner (1960), for instance, who advocated 'discovery learning' theory, indicating that this approach can make learning more effective as it is an active process that is stimulated through student curiosity. The teacher therefore devises situations, poses problems or questions, and creates the medium for the student to discover the structures and principles underlying the situation or topic area. This approach feeds into the currently advocated methods such as problem-based learning, which is an instructional method in which students work in small groups or individually to gain knowledge from simulated problem situations and acquire problem-solving skills at the same time.

Mentors can use these approaches in their learning facilitation roles. Problem-based learning can be implemented in the form of self-directed learning in clinical practice, in, for example, management of a staff conflict situation, management of a new illness or syndrome, the use of limited learning resources. The teacher, however, must ensure that the learning is directly linked to achieving learning outcomes or competencies identified in the module or the course.

Current definitions of teaching take these evolving learning philosophies into account. For example, according to Curzon (2003: 22), 'Teaching is a system of activities intended to induce learning, comprising the deliberate and methodical creation and control of those conditions in which learning does occur.' The definition thus does not reflect teacher-centred one-way information giving.

### Teacher-centred or learner-centred approaches

Teacher-centred teaching approaches clearly imply that the teacher directs the content of the teaching session. This may have advantages in being eco-nomical, in that with their deep knowledge of the subject the teacher can maximise the allocated time by selecting and focusing on the most significant areas of the topic.

Drawing on the theories underlying patient or service user–centred ther-apy for people with psychological problems, Rogers (1983) formulated the student-centred approach to learning, which formed a major landmark in approaches to teaching and learning. Rogers suggested that:

- Human beings have a natural potentiality for learning.
- Much significant learning is acquired through doing.
- Learning is facilitated when the student participates responsibly in the learning process.
- The most socially useful learning in the modern world is the learning of the process of learning, a continuing openness to experience and incorporation into oneself of the process of change.

## Activity 3.2    Teacher-centred or student-centred teaching

To follow up the aforementioned approaches to teaching, identify a number of factors that you consider to be the strengths and weaknesses of teacher-centred and student-centred teaching methods, in healthcare professional education programmes.

Jarvis (1995) notes that using teacher-centred methods of teaching reinforces hierarchical social relationships between teachers and learners (or mentor and student), and thereby replicates models of authority in which the teacher might be seeking to control and mould individuals to fit into social systems. Rogers (1983) suggested earlier that such approaches cause learners to become dependent on teachers and thereby obstruct growth and development.

The possible weaknesses of teacher-centred methods or strategies include the following:

- They assume that students usually lack discipline and are irresponsible.
- They disregard experience as a resource for learning.
- The orientation to learning is subject-centred rather than building on individual students' existing knowledge.
- The motivation to learn is external, for example by passing coursework.
- They can suppress the individual's creative powers.
- Students' opinions and questions tend to be largely overlooked.

Rogers sees the teacher as a facilitator of learning, a provider of resources for learning and someone who shares feelings as well as knowledge with learners. Furthermore, he indicates that crucial to effective facilitation of learning is the relationship between individual learners and the facilitator. The prerequisites for being an effective facilitator of learning are awareness of self and being oneself in the teaching situation, through (as mentioned briefly in Chapter 2):

- *Genuineness* – The facilitator portrays full honesty and willingness to declare their strengths and the areas in which they are lacking, where appropriate. They remain a real person and are not sucked into the image of a distant and authority-vested teacher.
- *Trust and acceptance* – The facilitator must be able to gain and retain the student's trust, and vice versa, and overtly accept any limitations students might have.
- *Empathic understanding* – The facilitator consistently endeavours to see situations from the learner's viewpoint.

Rogers contrasts the kind of learning that is concerned solely with cognitive functioning, for example acquiring knowledge, with that involving the whole person. The learning naturally needs to be guided by the approved curriculum for the course the student is on to be able to obtain the relevant award (i.e. qualification). Rogers suggests that it is possible for the teacher to build into a programme this freedom to learn. This can be done by using students' own experiences and problems so that relevance is more obvious, and by identifying relevant resources, both material and human, for their students. The goal of education is therefore to enable the student to become a fully functioning person as a whole (Rogers and Freiberg, 1994).

In healthcare learning, the student–centred approach is reflected in andragogy, but the latter needs to be tailored to individual students' responses to it. Facilitation of learning is also consistent with the andragogical approach to teaching and learning, as advocated by Knowles et al. (1998) (and discussed in Chapter 2) and with 'learning by insight', that is 'an unforeseen re-organisation by the learner of his field of experience' (Curzon, 2003: 83). A concept analysis of facilitation of learning by Cross (1996) revealed that the:

- prerequisites of being a facilitator are the facilitator's qualities of realness, that is, caring and empathy, access to learning situations and the motivation of students and social influences;
- defining attributes of facilitation are a process of enabling change, a climate of learning which includes mutual trust, acceptance and respect, and the nature of interaction being student centred, negotiated and collaborative;
- consequences of facilitation are reciprocal change and feedback, and increased independence.

---

## Activity 3.3   Mentoring Jane

Consider the following case study. Jane is a 34-year-old ex-schoolteacher who is now a first-year midwifery student. Jane is a graduate, who, after initial teacher training, soon found the job easy but had no wish to take on management responsibilities. The job was soon becoming too routine when she realised that in fact she had always wanted to be a midwife instead. Jane is also raising her own family and has remained an active member of the Parents and Teachers Association.

Consider the ways in which Jane's mentor, Julie, can take a learner-centred approach to learning facilitation during the practice placement. Make some notes taking into account Jane's previous vocation.

---

Mentors can consider ascertaining and adapting their facilitation of learning role to mentees' previous knowledge of health, and their preferred styles and approaches to learning, as noted in Chapter 2. Jane's age, responsibility and discipline as a qualified teacher and a mother can be taken into account when taking a learner-centred approach to placement learning. A self-directed approach to learning in consultation with Jane can be warranted.

Despite these benefits of the student-centred approach to teaching, there could also be drawbacks, some of which are identified in Box 3.1.

## Box 3.1 Arguments for, and criticisms of, the learner-centred or person-centred approach to teaching

**Arguments for:**

Motivates, as aims and objectives are clear and relevant.

Learning is meaningful.

Encourages divergent and critical thinking through dialogue.

Allows autonomy and creativity.

**Criticisms:**

Can be time consuming if emphasis is on how much ground is covered, rather than the nature of learning that occurs. (Rogers (1983) was aware of this, and suggested that there should be freedom within a system of constraints).

Structure and guidelines may suffer.

Timetables and deadlines might not get adhered to.

Assumption that everyone engages in self-directed learning.

Despite likely weaknesses, the student–centred approach to facilitation of learning is preferred as it entails more active involvement in learning. This is also consistent with old sayings such as, 'What we do we understand, what we see we remember, what we hear we forget' (Neary, 2000a: 93); and in relation to the senses and remembering, in that we remember 90 per cent of all we do, 50 per cent of all we see, but only 10 per cent of all we hear.

In experiential learning, as a way of adapting learning theories to methods of teaching, students need to be given opportunities for 'doing', that is, applying or using the knowledge or skill. For example, most healthcare courses include the topic 'moving and handling patients'. This is an apt example that lends itself to experiential learning, in that having been exposed to the knowledge base (e.g. principles of moving and handling), students can then learn by doing. This can occur in university skills laboratories under close supervision of the facilitator. Students can be given problem situations to solve, which could enable them to make the topic their own and internalise it.

A concluding suggestion on facilitation of learning is that, in the context of the current–day vehement push towards efficiency, mentors and mentees need to seize learning opportunities as they arise, which is also referred to as opportunistic learning or teachable moments.

## Facilitating Learners to Acquire Clinical Skills

Healthcare professions are skill-based vocations, which means that pre-registration education leads to becoming competent at performing specific clinical interventions to improve patients' or service users' health. Competence was defined and discussed in Chapter 2. According to Curzon (2003), a skill signifies having expertise in an activity which has been developed as the result of training and/or experience, enabling the individual to perform the particular task with effectiveness and flexibility. It requires effective mind and muscle co-ordination, resulting in the production of appropriate, swift and meaningful patterns of movement. These are the distinguishing features of a 'skilled activity', which also include dexterity, the ability to respond quickly, spatial ability, and the capacity to share attention among a number of more or less simultaneous demands (Curzon, 2003). These definitions and features apply to healthcare clinical skills, and competencies as well.

### Learning motor skills

Progression with learning and mastering clinical skills can be identified along a continuum that identifies early attempts at learning a skill to becoming proficient. A widely used framework for identifying levels of psychomotor skill development and testing in healthcare courses is that suggested by Steinaker and Bell (1979) in a taxonomy of experiential learning. The term *taxonomy* broadly refers here to levels of learning, that is, lower-level learning to higher levels. In Steinaker and Bell's model, skill development progresses from the lower-level exposure, through participation, identification and internalisation to dissemination.

Experiential learning refers to learning that involves going through the experience of actually doing or engaging in the skill. Competency or skill development through the different levels occurs over the three-year course. The five levels and the likely interpretation (or criteria) related to a clinical skill are presented in Box 3.2.

---

**Box 3.2   Taxonomy levels and criteria**

| Levels | Criteria |
|---|---|
| Exposure | Have some knowledge of concepts, terms and methods used in clinical practice<br>Show willingness to participate |

*(Continued)*

(Continued)

| Levels | Criteria |
|---|---|
| Participation | Interact well with patients/service users<br>Carry out activities under supervision<br>Explain activities when questioned |
| Identification | Apply theory to practice<br>Demonstrate awareness of situations<br>Interpret information correctly<br>Act on one's own without having to be prompted |
| Internalisation | Consistently apply theory to practice in a range of settings<br>Compare and contrast different approaches to practices<br>Determine implications of practices<br>Solve problems by analysis and evaluation<br>Show willingness to share experiences |
| Dissemination | Use opportunities to teach service users and families<br>Share experiences with peers and others<br>Accurately write and verbalise information about teaching and management issues |

Consider a mental health student who has to demonstrate a certain level of proficiency in helping or counselling skills by the end of their third year of professional education:

1   *Exposure* – refers to the student observing the mentor helping or counselling appropriate service users and becoming aware of the pre-conditions and specific helping skills being used by the mentor.
2   *Participation* – refers to when, under mentor supervision, the student attempts to use selected helping skills, e.g. low-level self-disclosure.
3   *Identification* – is when the student starts to feel competent at some of the helping skills, and this is acknowledged by their mentor.
4   *Internalisation* – can be difficult to achieve within the constraints of the pre-registration course, as this implies that the learner is so proficient at these skills that they see them as part of themselves as a person.
5   *Dissemination* – refers to being so knowledgeable and competent in a skill that the person can have specific and valid opinions about the skill, can explain them and even teach them, which is difficult to achieve in a pre-registration course.

To teach competencies at the appropriate level entails careful planning that determines the teacher's approach, student behaviour and assessment techniques. Another well-established model of learning a clinical skill is Benner's (2001) stages of skill acquisition, which is based on a framework initially deduced from how trainee pilots learn their vocations and eventually become experts in flying aeroplanes. These stages are novice, advanced beginner, competent, proficient and expert, in this sequence, and they relate to longer-term activities on expertise development as they progress from initial cruder attempts to more refined performance with a substantial associated knowledge base.

Fitts and Posner (1973) earlier suggested that there are three phases of learning a skill: the cognitive phase, associative phase and autonomous phase:

1  *Cognitive phase* – concerned with the learning of the procedure, but the more complex the skill, the longer the learning will take.
2  *Associative phase* – engaging in skilled performance of part-skills or in whole practical skills, and interfering responses are eliminated.
3  *Autonomous phase* – on the long-term the skill becomes automatic and can be performed without the student thinking much about it.

The three phases are not completely distinct, as they overlap, with one phase leading to the next.

## Teaching psychomotor skills

A major component of the mentor's role is to teach clinical skills. Various aspects need to be considered in relation to this.

### Activity 3.4    Skill acquisition and maintenance

Think of, and list all factors that a teacher needs to consider, and all preparations that they need to make to teach a particular clinical skill. Then list all factors that might affect efficient acquisition of the psychomotor skill in the practice setting. Finally, list all factors that might affect maintenance and performance of the clinical skill at the same or higher standard in practice settings.

There are several factors that need to be considered when preparing to teach a clinical skill. Those required for teaching blood glucose monitoring, for instance, include:

* which patient?
* condition requiring it;
* equipment needed;
* procedure for taking a blood sample;
* gain patient's consent;
* factors affecting reading of results;

- ensuring there's enough blood on the test strip;
- safety aspects;
- own knowledge;
- the student's knowledge base – practical and theoretical;
- result – up/down/normal;
- opportunities to practise;
- frequency of measurement;
- testing the equipment and cleaning it after use;
- evaluate, observe, supervise;
- what if !!
- time allocated;
- how to record competence.

A list of factors that need to be considered for a particular clinical activity like the one above is rarely fully prescriptive as there are other variables that need to be taken into account in relation to the individual patient's health problems or needs, and the equipment and other resources that are available.

Teaching a clinical skill requires first of all a skills analysis. Generally, the trust's procedure for the skill constitutes a very good basis for structuring a lesson plan for the skill. The mentor can also consider how the task is performed or executed, step-by-step, by those who are recognised as competent at that skill. These are discussed shortly. Such a detailed analysis of the clinical skill constitutes its performance criteria, which is discussed in Chapter 6. Box 3.3 presents a set of principles of teaching a skill or competency that stands the test of time (adapted from Curzon, 2003). These are generally fully used when teaching a skill in the HEI's skills laboratory, but can be easily adapted by the mentor when teaching in the practice setting.

---

## Box 3.3   Principles of teaching a skill or competency

1   *Initially demonstrate the skill in its entirety as a fully integrated set and cycle of operations.* The demonstration needs to be accompanied by a clear step-by-step commentary, and it must be a demonstration of mastery of the skill. The correct movements that go to make up the skill must be in evidence from the outset.

2   *Break the skill down into its component and subordinate activities.* Each action must be demonstrated, explained and analysed. The relation of separate activities to one another, and their integration into a hierarchy of sequences that make up the skill must be stressed.

*(Continued)*

*(Continued)*

3    *Skill acquisition lessons require supervised, reinforced and carefully spaced practice by students.* It is only by experiencing and repeating the essential movements that the learner can discover the kinaesthetic cues of successful performance.

4    *Continuous, swift and accurate feedback must be provided for the learner.* Delayed feedback on performance makes the feedback less effective.

5    *Assess part skills or the whole skill regularly and in realistic conditions.* Evidence should also be sought on the ability of the student to transfer the acquired skill to related situations.

6    *Achievement of competence at one level ought to be accepted as a necessary preparation for moving to higher level of skill.* The learner should be able to progress from competent performance to proficient, etc.

*Source*: Adapted from Curzon (2003)

The principles presented in Box 3.3 constitute a firm foundation for developing a skill-teaching session. Drawing on this, and on healthcare professionals' perceptions of factors that need to be considered when preparing to teach a psychomotor skill, the teacher should also consider taking the following actions before the actual skill-teaching session.

- Practise the skill yourself, using the relevant procedures and equipment.
- Ensure that, as teacher, you are up to date on grounds of evidence-based practice.
- Have all equipment and materials ready.
- Arrange for your learner(s) to hear and see.
- State the aim of the session.
- Show the finished product if possible.
- Ask the student/patient to verbalise the action.
- Arrange for the student/patient to practise the skill.

## Domains of learning and levels of skill acquisition

Precisely which components do healthcare students learn on their pre-registration courses? They learn knowledge and competence related to healthcare interventions. Each intervention comprises three domains of activity: psychomotor (skill), cognitive (knowledge) and affective (attitude) (e.g. Bloom, 1956; NMC, 2010a). The psychomotor domain refers to motor, muscular and co-ordination skills; the cognitive domain refers to the use of knowledge and information; and the affective domain refers to attitudes, emotions and values. The three domains equating broadly with skills, knowledge and attitudes, also equate largely with doing, thinking and feeling, respectively. The three domains are integrated essential components of each competency, and not necessarily distinct and separate activities. All healthcare interventions incorporate these three domains, and therefore learning the clinical skill must also incorporate all three components.

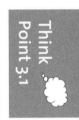

## Psychomotor, cognitive and affective domains of competencies

Consider any two clinical interventions (e.g. blood pressure taking, counselling, ward management, etc.) to ascertain whether each contains all three components: skill, knowledge and attitude.

**Think Point 3.1**

The sequence of events that both teacher and learner should engage in during skill acquisition is summarised in Table 3.1. It captures the principles of teaching and facilitation of learning of a psychomotor skill or competency that incorporates the cognitive and affective domains. The five components of the affective domain to be achieved by the learner are *receiving, responding, valuing, organising* and *characterising* (Krathwohl et al., 1999).

After practising the skill on several occasions, a summative assessment of competence will be performed by the mentor, and if the learner is deemed competent, he or she is usually permitted to practise the skill without direct supervision. One of the key purposes of Table 3.1 is to highlight how the cognitive and affective domains of learning are integral components of learning any clinical intervention. It involves taking a holistic approach and being aware of how the patient feels at all times during the activity.

As a general guide, 25 per cent of the lesson time should be used to demonstrate the skill, 15 per cent in verbal explanation and 60 per cent for guided practice. So, for effective acquisition of the skill or competency, it is important to consider the requirements for effective teaching. Other factors that affect effective and efficient acquisition of the skill include:

- the complexity of the skill;
- individual differences in speed of learning, or background;
- its transferability to real-life settings;
- teaching situation – environment, light, space, room temperature;
- the quality of instruction;

**TABLE 3.1**  Skills teaching sequence

| Psychomotor domain | Cognitive domain | Affective domain |
|---|---|---|
| Awareness that learner lacks the skill or is deficient in it ↓ | Establish learner's existing knowledge base underpinning the skill | Receiving – i.e. ensuring learner realises that it will be beneficial to learn the skill |
| Ensure the learner is motivated to learn the skill ↓ | Permit learner to be active in seeking related knowledge | Responding – learner is willing, and takes action to learn the skill |
| Analysis of the step-by-step procedure/components of the skill ↓ | Having clear objectives in learning the skill, and seek out possible sources of learning | Responding – learner appreciates the step-by-step procedure and the materials required at every step |
| Prepare equipments, etc. to teach the skill ↓ | Assembling appropriate equipment/devices and materials | |
| Demonstrate the skill at normal speed ↓ | Enable learner to observe and assimilate all details of the procedure | |
| Discuss each step just performed; re-demonstrate part skills as required ↓ | State rationale for each action; emphasise important points; discuss safety points; encourage learner to ask questions | Valuing – the rationales for each step taken; learner is willing to participate in performing the skill or part skill |
| Allow learner to perform whole skill/part-skills ↓ | Select components to work on, and actually 'doing' the skill, i.e. experiencing it | Organising – mental rehearsal of each skill component, with rationales; asking questions when unsure |
| Allow learner to perform the skill under supervision ↓ | Observe in silence, and with confidence in the learner | |
| Praise and review ↓ | Give feedback on performance. Reward progress. Correct any mistake. | Organising – reinforcement and sense of achievement, confidence |
| Allow to apply/repeat the skill under supervision | Using the learning in real situations. Assess progress and knowledge of rationales | Characterising – accepting the procedure is the correct way of performing the skill |

- knowledge of progress;
- availability of practice opportunities;
- availability of necessary equipment – checking them beforehand, describing them;
- getting feedback on skill performance;
- a positive approach;
- a running commentary if appropriate;
- a true-to-life setting;
- allowing time for discussion;
- time for practice – with positive reinforcement.

The types of knowledge associated with skills teaching is practical knowledge (i.e. 'knowing how') and theoretical knowledge (i.e. more in-depth 'knowing that'). Healthcare courses involve acquisition of both types of knowledge, and students are assessed on them at different academic levels, as detailed shortly in this chapter.

## Facilitating Knowledge Acquisition

Despite the current paradigm shift away from teaching to facilitation of learning, formal teaching also has its place in professional preparatory programmes. Many clinical skills and knowledge components are best imparted to learners through teaching. There will be times when the mentor will have to conduct short structured teaching sessions, probably in a room in the practice setting that can be used for this purpose. These sessions could be quite short or last an hour or more, delivered to a small group of learners or colleagues. Therefore a good insight into how to structure and deliver a teaching session is a useful component of the mentor's armoury of capabilities.

Effective teaching requires careful and thorough planning. The lesson needs to be structured fully, with flexibility built in depending on whether it is being delivered to a large group, or to smaller group workshops.

### Planning a structured teaching session

Logical sequencing of a structured teaching session constitutes lesson planning, an example of which is presented in Box 3.4.

---

### Box 3.4 Steps in lesson planning

1 Identify the topic of the lesson
2 Research the subject

*(Continued)*

*(Continued)*

3  Consider the students in relation to their previous knowledge
4  Write down the aims and objectives
5  Jot down as many points as possible in keeping with the objectives;
   then select, prune, sequence and structure these points
6  Select the appropriate teaching methods
7  Screen the activities against the objectives
8  Write the lesson (include teaching aids)
9  Prepare aids, equipment and classroom
10 Give the lesson
11 Evaluate the lesson

Each step presented in Box 3.4 requires specific attention in its own right. For instance, the third step requires the teacher to consider the students in relation to the knowledge they already have, as well as any prior reading that was required or suggested before the teaching session. This accords with the use of appropriate learning theories such as Ausubel et al.'s (1978) assimilation theory (discussed in Chapter 2). It is also consistent with Bruner's (1960) notion of linking new learning to previous knowledge.

As to the sequencing of lesson content (step 5 in Box 3.4), the Herbartian rule (Quinn and Hughes, 2007: 20) of sequence (or 'sequence procedures') for lesson presentation has stood the test of time and is also referred to as traditional rule. It involves proceeding from:

1  *The known to the unknown* – link new concepts to what is already known by the learner (e.g. water to blood, water pipes to blood vessels).
2  *The simple to the complex* – simple explanations to more complex areas; increasing level of complexity (e.g. diffusion in a jar to movement of oxygen and $CO_2$ between alveoli and alveolar capillaries; intra- and extra-cellular movement of potassium).
3  *The concrete to the abstract* – demonstrable link between visible components to invisible concepts (e.g. aspirates or infusion to acidity vs alkalinity).
4  *The particular to the general* – use specific examples to illustrate general theories (e.g. giving information reduces anxiety, people generally have a need to know what is happening).
5  *Observation to reasoning* – from how things are done to why.
6  *The whole view, to the parts, then return to the whole view* – the subject matter as an entity, analysis of component parts, return to the overall view.

Step 6 in Box 3.4 suggests selecting the appropriate teaching methods. A range of teaching methods is available to the teacher (see Box 3.5). The teaching method(s) selected for the session must be based on principles of teaching and on learning theories. The appropriateness of the method depends on the teacher's level of knowledge of theories and principles and their values, research and verbal skills, facilitative skills and on the aims of the lesson, for instance.

---

### Box 3.5   Most frequently used teaching methods

- Lectures
- Buzz groups/work in sub-groups
- Seminars
- Skills demonstration
- Guided study and open learning
- Role plays
- Problem-solving games/exercises/workshops
- Case study/patient-centred discussions

- Video recording a presentation
- Tutorial – individual/small group
- Ideas free flow exercises (previously known as brainstorming) e.g. concept-mapping
- Questions and answers
- Formal lessons
- E-learning and distance learning
- Group discussion
- Team teaching

---

Each of these methods has its advantages and disadvantages which are examined later in this chapter. The eighth step in Box 3.4 is to 'write the lesson', and includes identifying the teaching aids to be used. An example of a lesson plan is presented in Box 3.6.

---

### Box 3.6   Lesson or session plan

Date: ..............        Cohort: ..............        No. of students:  ......................

Title of the course/module:  ...............................

Subject of lesson:  ...............................................

*(Continued)*

*(Continued)*

Lesson aims:

Objectives:

Duration of lesson: ............................ (e.g. 1 hour)     Classroom: ........

| Time | Lesson content | Method | Teaching aids |
|---|---|---|---|
| 5 mins | Ascertain previous learning | Q & A* | – |
| 2 mins | State and explain lesson objective | Verbal exposition | PowerPoint slides |
| 10 mins | Concept I | Verbal exposition; Q & A | Whiteboard/ flipchart |
| 15 mins | Concept II | Verbal exposition; discussion | Whiteboard/ flipchart |
| 20 mins | Concept III | Students complete gapped handout; discussion | Gapped handout |
| 3 mins | Recapitulation, and recommend further reading | Verbal exposition | PowerPoint slides |
| 4 mins | Test and evaluation | Q & A | PowerPoint slides |
| 1 min | Announce title of next lesson + pre-reading | Verbal exposition | PowerPoint slides Written guidance on pre-reading |

*Q & A = Questions and answers

In relation to steps 8 and 9 in Box 3.4, or the use of an appropriate range of teaching aids such as whiteboard/flipchart or PowerPoint slides, some of these will be explained briefly, and their advantages and disadvantages will also be explored later in this chapter.

In planning the lesson, the teacher needs to consider likely constraints such as class size (for instance, is it 10 students or 200?), the number of pages of handouts if any given and availability of articles to be recommended as further reading. The teacher's aim in a lesson is to motivate, stimulate and communicate, to hold the class's attention and to achieve the defined objectives (Curzon, 2003), and therefore further essential considerations by the presenter are that:

1 The lesson must be pitched appropriately.
2 The teaching objectives must be realistic and clear.
3 Exposition must be ordered, simple and clear.
4 Development must be logical and sequential (flows coherently).
5 Presentation must be based on the essential 'social character' of the lesson (e.g. laboratory work or lecture).
6 Presentation must involve a variety of media.
7 Presentation must be related carefully to fluctuations in class attention.
8 Appropriate body language should be used.

Furthermore, a well-constituted presentation requires a clearly defined structure, the elements of which will normally include:

- An introduction, main part and conclusion.
- A logical sequence within each of the three parts.
- Regular sign-posting – this is where we have been, where we are now, and where we are about to go.
- Key learning points or main headings.
- Built-in monitoring and review – checking that the main learning points are being understood.

Appropriate communication and delivery skills are crucial. The presenter's role is also to engage with the audience, to challenge, to enthuse, to support, to motivate and to clarify. The next step is to give the lesson based on the lesson plan, and at the end of the lesson to evaluate it. The evaluation of the lesson can include use of an evaluation form, or to ask students to write three things they liked or found most useful about the session, aspects that can be seen as weaknesses, and suggestions for improvement.

## *Levels of theory acquisition*
The objective of many a teaching session is to impart knowledge and understanding of the designated topic area and, depending on various factors, it can

cover application, analysis and synthesis. These concepts are largely enshrined in the cognitive domain of Bloom's (1956) taxonomy of learning, which follows six hierarchical levels. The first or lower level of learning is the acquisition of knowledge, followed by the higher levels – comprehension, application, analysis, synthesis and evaluation, as illustrated here:

- *Knowledge* – refers to knowledge of topic area and content.
- *Comprehension* – refers to knowledge and comprehension.
- *Application* – refers to knowledge and comprehension, and application of concepts to general and specific settings.
- *Analysis* – refers to knowledge, comprehension, application and analysis of all components and alternative perspectives of each concept.
- *Synthesis* – refers to knowledge, comprehension, application, analysis and synthesis.
- *Evaluation* – refers to knowledge, comprehension, application, analysis, synthesis and evaluation (research, etc. on the topic).

*Knowledge* is the most basic level of learning, in which the student shows recall of specific facts, classifications, categories and sequences or methods in the topic area. It is a significant component of student assessment, as when the student has to demonstrate knowledge of human biology or of research methods. *Comprehension* refers to understanding and interpretation of the topic area, and can be shown by the student explaining theories and reasoning in their own words. It answers the question 'why' certain things happen or certain actions are taken, and the possible implications and consequences of these. *Application* occurs when the student applies knowledge and understanding to 'real-life' situations such as patient care. *Analysis* entails the ability to break down theories and concepts into their component parts, and explain the relationships between elements and the whole. It considers strengths and weaknesses, and separates the important aspects of information from the less important ones. *Synthesis* requires the individual to recombine various components of the topic area into a newly reconstructed whole. The student thereby utilises creativity in producing something unique, for example a plan, a design or a proposal. *Evaluation* implies the ability to make judgements regarding the value of material learned.

A simple and brief example of levels of learning related to 'the heart and blood pressure' is presented here to illustrate how cognitive levels of learning (Bloom, 1956) apply to learning in healthcare:

- *Knowledge* – knowing the anatomy and physiology of the heart and that pressure is exerted on the blood vessels each time the heart pumps a certain volume of blood through them.
- *Comprehension* – understanding that the reason for the heart beating rhythmically at approximately 60 beats every minute, generating a blood pressure (BP) of approximately 110/70 mm Hg is to ensure that essential ingredients such as glucose and oxygen are transferred to every tissue in the human body, and continuously.

- *Application* – awareness that the above BP reading can change for a variety of reasons, which might include diseased organs, and its significance for patient care.
- *Analysis* – when a person is seen to have high BP, the nurse needs to consider the whole range of reasons for this.
- *Synthesis* – designing, and advising the individual on, a set of actions to take to reduce their BP, and explaining the effects of unstable or high BP based on their unique aetiology and perceptions of high BP.
- *Evaluation* – ascertaining the value of the above set of actions, the skills and compliance of the patient in relation to them, and any research evidence on which actions are based.

The analysis of the cognitive domain of learning is essential as it involves critical analysis, which as already noted above entails breaking down information, exploring relationships between elements, or organisation and structure of information. Critical analysis involves the use of critical thinking, whereby we:

- Examine all the component parts of a situation.
- Identify what existing knowledge or information we have, related to the situation.
- Distinguish relevant information from irrelevant.
- Challenge generalisations, assumptions and rituals.
- Imagine and explore alternatives and choose appropriate options.

Gopee (2002b) discusses an effective way in which students can demonstrate critical analysis in their written assignments. Furthermore, more recently, Krathwohl (2002) has suggested a refinement of Bloom's (1956) level of knowledge acquisition by suggesting that the sequence be represented as follows:

1 Remember → 2 Understand → 3 Apply → 4 Analyse → 5 Evaluate → 6 Create

Krathwohl reverses the fifth and sixth levels, and this revised taxonomy is also a useful tool for identifying educational objectives, but, as with any new framework, it requires further work in its applicability to education programmes for healthcare professions.

## Teaching Methods and Teaching Aids

As discussed in the preceding section, skill demonstration is an effective way of teaching how to perform a professional skill. For structured lessons, effective teaching requires choosing and applying the appropriate teaching methods and aids, which are selected based on such factors as class size, aims of session, the students' existing knowledge levels and so on. The most frequently used teaching methods were identified in Box 3.5.

## Teaching methods – their advantages and disadvantages

Lectures remain an efficient teaching method for imparting knowledge and comprehension of a selected section of a subject area. A lecture is economical in that the knowledge can be imparted to hundreds of students by one lecturer during a particular teaching session. In fact, the lecture can be televised live to other lecture theatres in the same or other universities, even in other countries.

However, only a limited level of application and analysis can be achieved, as in very large groups it is difficult to cite examples of application to each student's field of interest. Moreover, it is easier for students to let their minds wander off the subject, which they generally can't do in smaller groups. Discussions, workshops and groupwork to explore application, analysis and synthesis of components of the lecture should therefore always follow lectures. Similarly, the advantages and disadvantages of other teaching methods also need to be appreciated.

### Optional activity – Teaching methods: Advantages and disadvantages

Taking an analytical approach, the strengths and weaknesses of each of the examples of different teaching methods listed in Box 3.5 can be identified. Consider these different teaching methods, and feel free to add others of your own, and identify as many advantages and disadvantages as you can for each of these methods.

You should have been able to identify one or two advantages and disadvantages of each of the aforementioned teaching methods. With *skill demonstration,* for instance, the advantages include visual display of the skill being performed. It reinforces previously acquired knowledge of the skill, activates many senses, enables procedure-directed practice, correlates theory and practice and is economical on time. The disadvantages could be that the learner might be left-/right-handed related to positioning of equipment, the skill might involve movements that are too complex, and too much information might be given. As learning and mastering a skill takes time, there is also a danger that the learner might be expected to perform the demonstrated skill at similar speed to the skilled demonstrator too soon.

The advantages of using *case studies* or *patient-centred discussions* as a teaching method are that there is active participation by students, that they are useful in the application of theory to practice, and that they present an opportunity for structured problem-solving. This increases understanding of the situation, diagnosing the problem, creating alternative solutions and predicting outcomes or implications. The disadvantages include insufficient patient data, extent of relevance for each student, etc.

## Presentation and teaching aids

There are several types of presentation aids that the teacher can utilise to vary the session, and thereby to retain the audience's attention or to add emphasis to aspects of the session. These aids include:

- flipchart and pens;
- whiteboard;
- PowerPoint slides;
- showing video-cassette or DVD recordings;
- plastic models of body parts/objects;
- gapped handouts;
- simulated materials or liquids.

The purpose of teaching aids is therefore to introduce variety into the teaching process, to extend sensory perception, to extend visual perception, to give meaning to abstractions and to assist in conceptualisation of complicated issues. The choice of visual aids involves consideration of appropriateness to the context or message, its cost-effectiveness, its availability and its suitability for your style of presentation. Each teaching aid requires a good understanding of how it works.

---

### Activity 3.5   Strengths and weaknesses of different teaching aids

Consider the strengths and weaknesses of the different teaching aids listed earlier, add other ones that you know of, and discuss with someone who has had some experience of classroom teaching what might be the strengths and weaknesses of each of these aids.

---

The *PowerPoint presentation* is a highly favoured method of presenting the knowledge base of a topic area to small or large audiences. The advantage is that it is prepared in advance and can be made very lively and colourful with pictures, cartoons and short films for more impact. The likely disadvantage might be that too many words are inserted in each slide, or if the slides are presented at a high speed this may not allow time for the audience to take the content in properly, or the equipment may fail (computers are known to explode).

## Issues with Facilitation of Learning in the Practice Setting

The mentor's role includes teaching mentees on a one-to-one basis, and at times in small groups in the practice setting. In both situations, the mentor needs to have a clear view of various components of the session, for example the content and sequence of the presentation, to ensure the learner gains an orderly, systematic understanding of the topic or clinical skill. However, the problematic situations that might arise when facilitating student learning may present challenges to the mentor.

For instance, there can be confusion in the interpretation of students' 'supernumerary status' during placements, in that the student may claim that they are there only to observe clinical activity, while the mentor believes that they should observe as well as participate. Supernumerary status can be manipulated by some students to the extent that they take excessive time off practice settings as study time, to the detriment of learning hands–on care and clinical skills, as many mentors claim that healthcare delivery is learned by doing, not by merely knowing about it. Perceptions of how to record reflective write-ups may vary. Differences of views or interpretation of rules need to be resolved by discussion and consulting appropriate educational or trust personnel for further guidance.

In facilitation of learning there can be differences in perception of what a reflective write-up is, how many words it should contain and whether to support arguments with references. In opportunistic learning, negotiating access to opportunities is a skill in its own right.

## Chapter Summary

This chapter has focused on the mentor's role in the facilitation of learning, both formal and informal, and has therefore examined:

- Whose learning healthcare professionals facilitate, and why; the various reasons for teaching; and the definitions and different perceptions of teaching, along with why healthcare professionals need to know how to facilitate learning.

- General perspectives on learning indicating a move away from teaching to the notion of facilitating learning. Approaches to teaching and learning, including teacher-centred methods, their uses and likely weaknesses, and the student-centred approach, which includes teaching styles and applying learning theories and styles. The movement comprises shifting away from formal teaching to much more learner-centred facilitation of learning.
- Facilitating learners to learn clinical skills, teaching a psychomotor skill, the domains of learning, levels of psychomotor skills and stages of skill acquisition.
- Facilitating knowledge acquisition, include undertaking planned and structured short teaching sessions, either on a one-to-one level, or in small groups of learners, or peers.
- The types of knowledge associated with skills such as practical knowledge and theoretical knowledge, along with levels of theory acquisition, and levels and stages of skill acquisition (taxonomy levels).
- Step-by-step planning of teaching sessions, including utilisation of different methods of teaching and teaching aids, and an analysis of how they can be used effectively.
- Some of the issues that might surface in the facilitation of learning in practice settings.

# Further Optional Reading

For a much more contemporary presentation and discussion on taxonomy of learning objectives, see:

- Anderson, L. and Krathwohl, D. (eds) (2001) *A Taxonomy for Learning, Teaching, and Assessing: A Revision of Bloom's Taxonomy of Educational Objectives* (2nd edn). New York: Merrill Press.

For a range of models of teaching, see:

- Biggs, J. and Tang, C. (2007) *Teaching for Quality Learning at University* (3rd edn). Maidenhead: Open University Press.
- Joyce, B., Calhoun, E. and Hopkins, D. (2009) *Models of Learning: Tools for Teaching* (3rd edn). Maidenhead: Open University Press.

# 4

# The Practice Setting as an Effective Learning Environment

## Introduction

Having explored the concept of mentorship in Chapter 1, perspectives, theories and styles of learning in Chapter 2, and facilitation of learning in Chapter 3, this chapter focuses on the factors that make health and social care settings effective learning environments. Ensuring that the practice setting has an effective learning environment is a key role of the mentor according to research (e.g. Darling, 1984; Phillips et al., 2000), and under the domain 'Create an environment for learning' the NMC (2008a: 55) indicates that the mentor should be competent in creating 'an environment for learning, where practice is valued and developed, that provides appropriate professional and inter-professional learning opportunities and support for learning to maximise achievement for individuals'.

This chapter therefore examines the nature of effective learning environments in practice settings, ways in which healthcare professionals can be involved in creating, maintaining and monitoring such environments, educational policies, along with the issues related to student practice placements. Other aspects related to learning environments are identified under the domain 'Context of practice', and managing change, which are analysed in Chapter 5.

## Chapter outcomes

On completion of this chapter, you should be able to:

1   Clearly identify the reasons for healthcare profession students requiring practice placements.
2   Recognise the reasons for ascertaining students' clinical experiences that meet their learning needs, and ascertain students' own perspectives, hopes and expectations before the start of placements.
3   Identify how a functional learning ethos can be created and maintained in the practice setting, including research findings, inter-professional learning, and annual education audits of practice placement settings as components.
4   Identify the benefits of work-based learning as a concept and activity in its own right, and the utilisation of learning pathways.
5   Identify guidelines, policies and standards for learning environments, and how practice settings can become learning organisations.
6   Recognise the likely problematic aspects of practice placements, such as with integration of theory and practice, and with supernumerary status, and the likely solutions to these.

# Students on Practice Placements

This section of the chapter explores why practice placements are required, and students' perspectives, hopes and expectations in relation to practice objectives and clinical experiences during placements.

## The requirement for practice placements

The key reasons for practice settings having to be learning environments for student practice placements are as follows. First, healthcare professions comprise skill- or competency-based activities, and these skills are acquired predominantly in practice settings. Several hundred student nurses, numerous AHP and medical students start their pre-registration or pre-service courses each year, and each student requires practice placements in practice settings to learn patient care skills directly, or to consolidate and extend their learning from university skills laboratories. Most suitable practice settings in the local trusts and the independent sector are used for placements, and the placement of all these students is arranged by the education institution's placement department. Each practice setting is advised in advance of which students are starting on placement with them, and when. Students arrive on placement with a set of practice competencies to be achieved during the placement, which need to be planned in accordance with the specialist clinical skills and knowledge that the particular setting offers.

Furthermore, the NMC's (2008a) competence for mentors under 'creating an environment for learning' comprises the following outcomes:

- Support students to identify both learning needs and experiences that are appropriate to their level of learning.
- Use a range of learning experiences, involving patients, clients, carers and the professional team, to meet defined learning needs.
- Identify aspects of the learning environment which could be enhanced, negotiating with others to make appropriate changes.
- Act as a resource to facilitate personal and professional development of others.

Another reason for practice settings needing to be learning environments is the increasingly popular concept of work-based learning (discussed later in this chapter), which clearly recognises the wide occurrence and value of learning in practice settings. However, various research studies have in the past revealed weaknesses of practice settings as learning environments. Consequently, for learning to occur, the practice setting must embody an ethos that nurtures and supports learning, and does not deter it.

### Students' perspectives, hopes and expectations

A number of practice settings have an established welcome and orientation programme for students starting practice placement with them, and an induction pack with specific clinical objectives for new qualified healthcare professionals. A named mentor is allocated to each student prior to the start of the placement, along with associate mentors. Both the mentor and the mentee have certain hopes and expectations of each other. So what does the student anticipate encountering at the start of the placement?

---

## Activity 4.1    Student expectations from the placement

Your work base clearly has a wide range of specific knowledge and competence to offer learners during practice placements. From your experience of having students on placement, make some notes on what you feel are the expectations that students might have on starting placement in your practice setting.

---

In addition to students' expectations, the staff in the practice setting naturally also have certain expectations of students. They hope the student will be punctual, make every effort to integrate with the team, and be open-minded about the way care is delivered in the particular practice setting. The mentor might expect the student to seek out learning experiences and opportunities, and ask questions about aspects that they do not understand. Box 4.1 lists some of the characteristics of 'good' learners that were identified by student mentors.

---

### Box 4.1    Significant characteristics of learners for effective learning

- Keen, enthusiastic and motivated to learn
- Open-minded
- Identifies own learning needs
- Open to feedback and constructive comments
- Is punctual
- Reflects on experiences
- Knows own limitations
- Able to adapt to different practice settings
- Does not have negative thoughts prior to start of placement
- Utilises learning opportunities
- Communicates effectively
- Wants to self-improve
- Reads round the subject area

---

### Advanced preparation of learners

Students find it useful if, prior to the practice placement, the practice setting sends out a welcome letter, and even asks the student to come for an informal pre-placement visit. It is useful if the student can also be advised of any recommended preparatory reading related to the clinical specialism. This action is in line with Ausubel et al.'s (1978) concept of 'advanced organiser', which suggests that learning is likely to occur more effectively if new experiences are linked to prior knowledge.

The value of communication prior to the beginning of the placement is that the student begins to become familiar with the practice setting, gets to know more about the clinical specialism, meets the mentor, and staff get to know the student as well. The aim of this would be to ensure that the clinical experiences that the student will encounter meet their learning needs and enable the achievement of their practice objectives.

## Creating and Maintaining a Learning Ethos in the Practice Setting

Healthcare students acquire knowledge and competence at universities which are seen as well-established learning environments. The value of work-based learning (WBL) in enabling healthcare practitioners to achieve fitness to practise was referred to briefly in Chapter 1. However, to what extent are practice settings learning environments?

---

## Activity 4.2    A learning ethos in the practice setting

Using your current and past experience of factors that are significant in creating an effective learning experience for students during practice placements, make notes on the following: Who are the key people who are role models for learners (pre- and post-registration, other) in practice settings? What are the factors that are important for the creation of a positive learning environment (including research-based factors) for everyone within any particular practice setting?

---

To be a role model for anyone can be a sobering prospect for most people. In response to who the role models in practice settings are, you would have identified a range of qualified healthcare professionals and probably even some unqualified staff involved in practice-based learning, including:

- everyone acting as a mentor;
- ward sisters/charge nurses;
- team leaders;
- specialist nurses (e.g. pain specialists);
- PEFs;
- other RNs on pay bands 5 to 8;
- allied healthcare professionals (e.g. physiotherapists, occupational therapists);
- tutors;
- other students;
- senior doctors, mainly consultants;
- outreach workers;
- clinical managers;
- healthcare assistants, for specific skills;
- everyone who works in the practice area.

The concept of role models was examined in Chapter 1.

## Practice settings as learning environments

In response to Activity 4.2, that is, identifying the factors that are important for the creation of a positive learning environment, you might have noted friendly staff, positive attitude and allocated time for teaching. Good communication is of course essential, as is the learner feeling that they are part of the team. Team members with up-to-date knowledge of the latest research in their specialism generally make a positive impression. The availability and accessibility of research literature in the working environment, stocked in a learning resources section or in a resource room, also creates a positive image.

Furthermore, you might have noted that staff showing some awareness of students' likely learning needs and their stage of knowledge and competence development also creates positive impressions. The enthusiasm of team members with responsibility for teaching in practice settings, and PEFs' input, generate impetus for learning. Constructive comments on skill performance in an appropriate environment are usually appreciated by learners. A culture in which clinical staff are open to new ideas and share new learning from courses also presents healthy perspectives, as does good staff morale.

Numerous research studies have been conducted on the effectiveness of practice settings as learning environments over the years, and new research in this area continues as the dynamics in practice settings evolve. A study by Newton et al. (2009), for instance, revealed that a supportive social and cultural arena that enables the student to become part of the clinical team is very important.

However, in an earlier landmark study of practice learning environments, Fretwell (1980) aimed to find out:

- Whether students felt that they needed teaching in the ward environment.
- The attitudes of trained staff and learners as to the amount of teaching that might be needed.
- Who should teach?

In conclusion, Fretwell identified the key components of the 'ideal learning environment' as anti-hierarchy, teamwork, negotiation, communication and availability of trained nurses for responding to students' questions.

The first aim of the study was to explore whether student nurses felt that they needed teaching in the ward environment – because in the 1980s nursing students were rostered and salaried employees, and their employee status usually took precedence over learning. This changed when students were given supernumerary status in the early 1990s, and a bursary of approximately half of their salary. However, the public services union, UNISON (2006), has been urging the government to scrap the bursary system for student nurses and pay them a 'decent wage' instead. The union's researchers found that 61 per cent of students were taking extra paid employment to supplement their income, and most of them acknowledged that this had a detrimental effect on their learning. Many students were in debt, 14 per cent of them owing more than £10,000. Two out of five students in the survey said that they had seriously considered withdrawing from the course because they had to take extra employment.

This movement began in around 2004, and on behalf of UNISON, Harrison (2005) suggests that giving students more money can be achieved without ending students' supernumerary status. A report in *Nursing Standard* (Anon., 2006) indicated that a £10,000-a-year bursary was being recommended for a nursing student.

In addition to Fretwell's research, a number of other studies were conducted during the 1980s to establish the factors that make practice settings good or effective learning environments. One of these was Orton's (1981) study, which concluded by identifying the characteristics of wards that showed High Student Orientation and those that reflected Low Student Orientation. In High Student Orientation wards respondents stated, for instance:

- 'All staff treated students with kindness and understanding and showed willingness to teach us.'
- 'Everyone got on well.'
- 'Each patient had individual total care however long it took.'
- 'Every nurse was made to feel important.'

On the other hand, in Low Student Orientation wards, 96 per cent of students said that they learnt more from other students than from qualified staff, and that:

- 'The atmosphere was not very relaxed which made you worry about asking questions.'
- 'The ward sister did not respect us at all and gave us ten jobs to do at once.'

---

## Activity 4.3   Creating a learning ethos in the practice setting

1  Consider the findings and recommendations of the research studies just discussed.
2  Do an itemised summary of your own identifying factors that make a good learning environment.
3  How far does your own practice setting meet with the recommendations and factors that you've identified?
4  Identify areas in which your practice setting is weak or could benefit from further improvement.

---

The responses to studies on practice learning environments could be categorised as factors that promote learning in the practice setting, and those that hinder, a number of which are identified in Box 4.2.

## Box 4.2   Factors that promote learning and those that hinder learning in the practice setting

**Factors that promote learning**

- Registrants' level of knowledge of their clinical specialism
- Adequate time to teach
- Practical demonstration of skills
- Students feeling that they can take their time to practise the skills
- A learning ethos
- Teaching on a one-to-one basis
- Adequate staffing levels
- Adequate planning and preparation
- Supporting learning resources and information
- Approachable staff

**Factors that hinder learning**

- Interruptions
- Over-busy ward area
- Lack of time
- Staff, patient and learners' attitudes
- Standards of equipment
- Not enough information communicated
- Learner–staff ratio too high
- Inadequate staffing levels
- Student disinterested
- Disorganised programme of teaching
- Poor leadership

For non-hospital areas such as primary care settings, Gopee et al. (2004) make the following recommendations for enhancing these as learning environments:

- Mentor–mentee matching in accordance with seniority of practitioner and the student's particular learning needs.
- Management support to enable designated time to be given for mentoring, so that students and mentors feel time spent in this way is valued by their seniors.
- Raised awareness of the need to integrate theory and practice.
- Ensuring student practice outcomes are achievable, for example carrying out dressings might not be available in, say, placement with school nurses.
- Prior notices of placement and appropriate timing, for example not allocating student to school nursing placement during school holidays.
- Ongoing professional development for all grades of staff, for example in Professional Development Units.
- More effective communication at all levels, and trust–university–mentor partnership.
- All mentors (and practice teachers) ensuring that they maintain the relevant NMC's standards.
- Access to clinical supervision for all qualified staff.

In another study on practice learning environments, Wood (2005), for example, reports on the experiences of a group of pre-registration mental health nursing students during practice placements, which indicated that they experience 'conflicting pressures', while their mentors experience difficulty supporting them because of high clinical workload.

Mikkelsen Kyrkjebø and Hage (2005) report on a Norwegian study examining nursing students' development of new knowledge in clinical practice and of healthcare processes, cross-professional collaboration and the handling of adverse events. The findings suggest a deficiency in improvement in knowledge in clinical practice and the existence of a theory–practice gap. The authors recommend a change in the culture within healthcare and health professional education to utilising learning models that encourage reflection, openness and scrutiny of underlying individual and organisational values and assumptions.

Henderson et al. (2006) report on an Australian study exploring students' perceptions of psychosocial support available in practice learning environments. They found that the medium for developing mentor–mentee relationships and students feeling part of the team were significant factors in enhancing student learning during practice placements. Henderson et al. (2010) later explored the organisational culture of practice settings that influence learning, which they discuss under the headings:

- Recognition of learners and learning in the organisation
- Accomplishment, i.e. acquisition of new knowledge and skills
- Affiliation, i.e. feeling part of the organisation, the team in the practice setting
- Influence, i.e. feeling safe to express opinions and suggest ideas

These more contemporary study findings relating to mentors' workload, theory–practice gap, organisational values and psychosocial support reflect different issues to those identified earlier by Fretwell (1980) and Orton (1981). Based on the above accounts of the subject area, a clinical learning environment can be defined as a practice setting that manifests a psychosocial ethos and culture, with related supportive resources, that fosters mutual learning amongst all healthcare professionals, learners and clientele, and where care and treatment are founded on evidence-based practice. The recommendations from earlier and recent studies regarding aspects that constitute good and effective learning environments form key components of educational audits.

## Educational audit of practice placement settings

After Fretwell's and Orton's research, later studies on practice learning environments (e.g. Rotem and Hart, 1995) focused more directly on exploring the factors that can be identified as criteria in educational audit tools to monitor the suitability of practice settings for student placement. The criteria for suitability include evidence of a systematic approach to care delivery and holistic care (and the practice setting's philosophy of care). Orton et al. (1993), for instance, specifically focused on educational auditing, and asked qualified staff and students the same questions separately, in relation to:

1   orientation to the placement;
2   theory and practice;
3   supernumerary status;
4   staff attitudes and behaviour;
5   the mentor;
6   progressive assessment.

Using questionnaires, under 'orientation to the placement', for instance, they asked qualified staff:

1   Do staff make students feel welcome on arrival?
2   Are students shown round the ward?
3   Are students allocated a mentor in their first week?
4   Etc.

Correspondingly, they asked students:

1   Did staff make you feel welcome?
2   Were you shown round the ward?
3   Were you allocated a mentor in your first week?
4   Etc.

Thus, having gathered data on the views of key players, Orton et al. (1993) then designed an education audit tool with specified standards for placement areas. It is an NMC requirement that annual educational audits are carried out for each practice setting where students are placed for learning clinical skills. Under the headings used by Orton and colleagues to explore the suitability of practice settings as learning environments there are a number of 'ward learning climate indicators'.

Newton et al. (2010) go a step further by empirically testing their 'Clinical Learning Environment Inventory' which comprises 42 criteria grouped under six sections, namely: personalisation, student involvement, task orientation, innovation, satisfaction and individualisation. They conclude their test by suggesting modifications to the inventory, and by recommending further research to establish the consistency of the modified inventory, which implies that even in 2010, the best educational audit tool has not yet been established.

## Activity 4.4   Strengths and weaknesses of your work base as a learning environment

The Orton et al. (1993) report contains the 'Ward Learning Climate Indicators' questionnaire used in the study. See if you can locate the publication from a university library and, if you can, then using the items in the qualified staff section, mark your own practice setting in one of the four boxes for each item.

Alternatively, the actual items on the educational audit form used at your healthcare trust in partnership with the university can be similarly used. A copy of the current completed audit form is usually lodged in the practice setting as a paper copy or electronically. This exercise will highlight areas of strengths in, and where improvements can be made to, your own practice setting as a learning environment. Can you do anything about the weaker points? In fact, can you devise a SMART (specific, measurable, achievable, realistic and time-limited) action plan to make tangible improvements to the weaker areas (learning climate indicators' or audit criteria)?

Each university devises its own research-informed educational audit tool in collaboration with the local healthcare trusts. The educational audit form constituted jointly by one of the UK Strategic Health Authorities and a local university comprises 20 standards (or criteria) related to:

1   Management of practice area
2   Learning and teaching opportunities
3   Assessment of practice
4   Effective resources
5   Quality and evaluation of practice

Examples of standards criteria under 'Management of Practice Area', for instance, are:

- A philosophy of care is used that reflects core values of patient-centred planning and delivery of care.
- The provision of care reflects patient privacy, dignity, religious and cultural beliefs and practices.

Evidence needs to be available to demonstrate how each criterion is achieved. The educational audit document includes a section for recording the qualifications of each member of staff, of particular significance being which part of the profession's regulatory body's register they are on, and also whether they have a mentoring qualification and have been attending annual update sessions on mentoring. Other post–registration qualifications are also recorded. Box 4.3 shows the content of another section of the audit form that contains key information that identifies the particular practice setting.

---

## Box 4.3    Placement details

XXX UNIVERSITY, NURSING, MIDWIFERY and HEALTHCARE
Multi-Professional Practice Environment Profile

Name of Trust/Organisation:

Site Location/Address:

Name of Ward/Department Unit/Organisation:

Telephone No:

Email address:

Name of Placement Contact:

Type of Service Provision:

Date of Review:

Date of Previous Review:

Names of Reviewer/Review Team:

Name of Academic Link:

    Practice Education Facilitator:
    Practice Facilitator:
    Clinical Educator:

Name of Academic Institutions Placing Students

    University:
    College of Further Education:
    Other:

Work Patterns, e.g. length of shift patterns:    am:

                pm:

                Night:

---

Naturally, each item in this section of the audit form is important. The form also has a section for clinical staff to identify and list all the formal and informal teaching and learning opportunities that are available in the particular practice setting.

---

### Activity 4.5    Formal and informal learning opportunities

Identify and make two lists, one of all the formal learning opportunities that are available in your own practice setting, and one of the informal ones. You might find it useful to discuss the activity with a colleague in the same practice setting.

---

For formal learning, you might have mentioned lectures by the clinical nurse specialist, for instance; and for informal learning opportunities you might have mentioned when you explain to the learner why the doctor has changed a patient's medication. There are likely to be various teaching and learning opportunities in your work-base setting. Maybe one of the consultants holds regular formal teaching sessions for junior doctors, which all health professionals in the particular area are welcome to attend. Maybe pharmaceutical or medical devices company representatives give talks and demonstrations on their products in the practice setting. Further examples of teaching and learning opportunities that tend to be identified when completing educational audit forms are presented in Box 4.4.

---

### Box 4.4    Formal and informal learning opportunities

**Formal teaching**

- Lectures by senior doctors
- Assessment-related teaching
- Interviews – initial, halfway and final
- Teaching while carrying out patient care, i.e. work-based learning
- Setting students' learning tasks

**Informal learning opportunities**

- Learning from patient with new condition
- Change in patient's condition discussed at handover
- Asking questions informally
- Reflection-in-action and reflection-on-action
- Informal chat in the staff room during coffee break

**Formal teaching**

- Practice development manager's guidance
- Teaching by PEFs
- Cascade trainers
- In-service/postgraduate training
- Observing RNs, physiotherapists and other AHPs, or doctors performing clinical skills

**Informal learning opportunities**

- Updating procedures and clinical guidelines' folders and learning resources
- Access to computer databases

If preferred, the resources for learning available in the practice setting can be grouped as human and non-human resources. Formal learning opportunities, such as teaching sessions and skill demonstrations, require human resources and include inter-professional learning. Non-human resources include printed instructions on how to use equipment, learning about medications, ventilator monitors or behaviour therapy. Many of the resources needed to deliver patient care can also be used for learning and for achieving clinical and managerial objectives. Other learning resources include a room that can be used for teaching and learning, with internet-enabled computers, whiteboard or flipcharts, for instance. The learning resource files compiled by clinical staff as part of projects or course assignments are also usually available for consultation and learning.

## Inter-professional learning

As for inter-professional learning (IPL) in practice settings, the concept is promoted in various authoritative documents (e.g. DH, 1999, 2001c; UKCC, 1999; NMC, 2008a). Successful education programmes and projects (e.g. DH, 2008b; Goldsmith et al., 2009) are documented on the internet and presented at conferences.

The basis for IPL is multi-professional working, in that to resolve the individual patient's or service user's health problem (or to avert it), a group of different healthcare professionals such as nurses, doctors, dieticians, physiotherapists and speech and language therapists input their own areas of professional expertise as appropriate. Multi-professional working can involve different healthcare professionals attending to the patient, delivering their clinical input and withdrawing. These actions can be fragmented and inadequately co-ordinated and recorded. Inter-professional working implies better co-ordinated patient care with fuller communication, verbal and written, between different healthcare professionals. Inter-professional learning extends the concept to the exchange of knowledge, understanding and clinical skills. Lloyd (1999) and Pirrie et al. (1998) also distinguish similarly between multi-disciplinary working and inter-disciplinary working.

IPL also comprises informal and formal learning. Informally, for instance, the nurse explains to the occupational therapist the plan of care for a particular patient and the rationales for each action. In turn, the occupational therapist designs a plan of action and explains the rationales from their perspective. This could also form the basis for work-based learning, which is explored in detail shortly.

Formal IPL involves attending structured learning programmes, such as courses that are designed for specified healthcare professionals, covering the physical, social and psychological basis for health and illness and the clinical skills that aid recovery. Some courses (or part of them) are designed for shared learning by, say, nursing and medical students (e.g. Freeth and Nicol, 1998; Reeves and Pryce, 1998; Morrison et al., 2004). Others, such as a course on counselling, might be designed for nurses, social workers and specific allied health professionals.

Informal IPL refers to all modes of unstructured, incidental or opportunistic teaching and learning between different professional groups, while inter-professional education (IPE) refers specifically to university-designed courses that result in students being awarded diplomas or degrees. In their study of 'multi-professional education', Pirrie et al. (1998: 415) use the term to describe 'a range of situations in which students from different health and social care professions come together to enhance their understanding of particular elements of their professional practice'. They conclude that there are considerable benefits associated with multi-professional education in healthcare, although it needs to be adequately resourced, and its success depends on the commitment of all staff involved.

Inter-professional education is defined by the Centre for Advancement of Interprofessional Education (CAIPE) (2010: 1) as follows: 'Interprofessional education occurs when two or more professions learn with, from and about each other to improve collaboration and the quality of care.' It indicates that IPE includes such learning in academic and work-based settings before and after qualifying. Alternatively, IPL is a more holistic term that encompasses all manner of inter-professional learning, while IPE refers specifically to learning by students on formal courses.

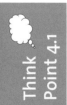

**Think Point 4.1**

## IPL and IPE

Consider to what extent IPL occurs in your work setting. In those settings where it does occur, is it linked to IPE?

Inter-professional learning has been explored for some time as either IPL, IPE or shared learning, by, for example, Long et al. (2001) and Miller et al. (1999). A report by Hughes and Marsh (2006) for the Creating an Inter-professional Workforce programme presents a structure for implementing inter-professional working, which also identifies a number of themes and issues related to IPL.

In a study of post-qualified students undertaking an inter-professional studies programme, Salmon and Jones (2001: 18) found that skilful facilitation of learning was particularly important, and involved gaining an 'understanding of the knowledge bases, aspirations and values that underpin those (healthcare professions') roles'. Some of the issues related to IPL are as follows.

Hean et al. (2006) report on a study which concluded that different AHP students saw themselves as distinct from other professional groups. This is healthy as it enables them to establish their professional identity prior to exploring commonalties between them. However, when they identified the characteristics that made them different, for example physiotherapy students indicating that they believe that being a team player made them different, other groups also stated having this characteristic. This suggests that many of the characteristics of each AHP group are probably very similar. Naturally, their areas of clinical expertise have different focuses. Reeves and Pryce (1998) found that medical, dental and nursing students revealed inconsistencies in their stereotypical attitudes towards the status of their intended professions. The authors suggest that these observations provide early evidence of key cultural, professional and institutional issues that need to be considered in planning and implementing inter-professional curricula.

Education programme planners need to be aware of the issues with IPE just highlighted so that they can make relevant adjustments to retain teaching effectiveness. However, healthcare learners benefit from IPL. One way that the care and treatment of particular patients are planned and delivered inter-professionally is through integrated care pathways. These in turn can form the basis for constituting learning pathways for students.

Additionally, as for inter-professional assessment of clinical (or practice) skills, this can be implemented to a certain extent, bearing in mind the concept of 'due regard', which the NMC (2008a) uses to indicate that summative assessment of competence can only be legitimately performed by a mentor whose name is in the same part of the NMC's register as the mentee, i.e. in the same field of practice. Holt et al. (2010: 264), for instance, report on a project that explored ways of assessing communication, team working and ethical practice, which are three essential competences for all health professionals at five HEIs and in 16 professional groups in the UK. They took into account the stance of professional statutory and regulatory bodies, practice-based and academic staff and service users and carers on assessment of these skills, and report that multi-professional assessment is feasible in the endeavour to 'accurately and fairly measure capabilities to help students develop into proficient and effective practitioners' (2010: 264).

## Utilising learning pathways

The student's placement could in many settings beneficially incorporate patient journeys and patient care pathways that are concepts identified by the Department of Health (e.g. 2002a, 2009). 'Care maps', 'collaborative care pathways', 'multi-disciplinary pathways of care', are all terms that are used interchangeably. Once the care pathway for a particular patient has been formulated, it can be included in the student's learning pathway whereby the student can gain knowledge of the interventions and underpinning rationales undertaken to enable the patient to recover from their health problem. The student's learning can be supplemented by pre-arranged lectures and workshops held at the university or within healthcare trusts, and by self-directed study.

In *Liberating the Talents,* the Department of Health (2002a) notes that 90 per cent of patient journeys begin and end in primary care. The Department of Health (2004b: 1) defines a patient pathway as 'the route that a patient will take from their first contact with a NHS member of staff (usually their general practitioner [GP]), to the completion of their treatment. It also covers the period from entry into a hospital or a Treatment Centre, until the patient leaves.' The word *integrated* is added to care pathways to signify inter-disciplinary input.

The definitions of care pathways include that by Overill (1998: 93), who suggests that integrated care pathways provide 'locally agreed, multi-disciplinary practise-based guidelines and evidence where available, for a specific client group'. Care pathways specifically designed for particular illnesses are well documented in healthcare literature. Examples of this include van Wijngaarden et al. (2006) on thrombolysis in acute ischaemic stroke, McNicholl et al. (2006) on the care of dying patients, and Bowker et al. (2005) on the Type-1 diabetes mellitus. Several care pathways are also available on the Department of Health's website (e.g. DH, 2008c).

Research on care pathways includes an exploration of the application of Goldberg and Huxley's Pathway to Care by Issakidis and Andrews (2006) (in Australia), which revealed that being aged over 55 years or living in a rural area was associated with less access to certain healthcare sectors such as outpatient care. An evaluation of the application of the Liverpool Care Pathway

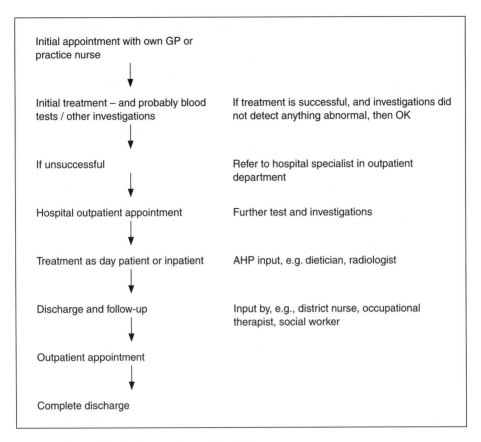

**FIGURE 4.1**  A patient's journey through healthcare

for the dying patient indicates that the pathway made patient care clearer and uncomplicated, with specific methods of assessment and measurement of symptoms and outcomes (McNicholl et al., 2006).

The focus on patient journey approach was also evaluated by Baron (2009), for instance, who found various benefits of this approach, including greater patient involvement in their recovery from illness and more effective inter-professional working.

A student on practice placement could encounter a patient whose journey through healthcare is taking them along the pathway identified in Figure 4.1.

The DH (2009) identifies the patient pathway for an adult visiting their GP with alcohol-related problems, whereupon, following a systematic set of actions, an alcohol treatment pathway is devised for him or her, a journey that includes all the stages that lead up to treatment, including outpatient consultations and diagnostic tests and procedures. Integrated care pathways continue with the care and treatment required by the patient to the point of maximum recovery from the health problem.

The student can follow a patient's care pathway through the healthcare system closely to gain knowledge and understanding of the care and treatment required in particular illnesses. The student's learning pathway through the practice placement would involve exposure to, and engagement with, selected patient care pathways, supplemented in various ways, for example by practice-based teaching by the mentor and other health professionals.

HEIs work in collaboration with local trust clinicians to develop and implement learning pathway programmes in healthcare course curricula, based on patient journeys, with web-based scenarios for students to investigate. A suitable definition of learning pathways related to healthcare students' learning is difficult to locate. Essentially, a learning pathway constitutes a selection of integrated care pathways for patients with different health problems that will enable the student to attain comprehensive learning about patient or service user care and treatment in the particular specialism, and achieve identified placement objectives. Furthermore, as care pathways incorporate involvement of an appropriate combination of nursing or midwifery, medical, social work and AHP staff, learning pathways are increasingly being referred to as 'inter-professional learning pathways'.

Pollard and Hibbert (2004) report on a project on enhancing student learning using patient pathways, and conclude that patient pathways constitute one way of turning students' learning during practice placements from an *ad hoc* set of activities into logical and organised experiences. Using patient pathways therefore offers a more structured approach to learning as opposed to relying on unplanned, opportunistic, and therefore erratic, learning.

The learning pathway for a student on an Emergency Department placement could include the student starting with a day with the ambulance services, following a patient with a suspected fracture to the X-ray department, spending time working with plaster technicians, and so on. Furthermore, if the same patient also suffers from alcohol- or drug-related problems, for example, or displays aggressive or even violent behaviour, these themselves present instances for further learning for the student, the management of which can be explored up to maximum recovery.

Learning pathways have been identified as beneficial by Hutchings and Sanders (2001), for instance, who describe a successful project in which the development of learning pathways achieved its aims, which were to improve the quality of learning as well as being enjoyable, and promoting high-quality patient care. Students and clinical staff worked in partnership and had equal responsibilities for improving the quality of learning.

The effectiveness of learning pathways in making learning more comprehensive was also explored by Anderson (2009), for instance, who conducted a qualitative study, which revealed that the use of learning pathways enable students to develop 'a greater awareness and understanding of the delivery of healthcare in primary care settings and they expanded their nursing knowledge and skills' (2009: 835). However, she also notes that some students felt that learning pathways fragmented their learning in the base placement area. The fragmentation of learning downside needs to be heeded as the subjects of Anderson's study were final placement student nurses who felt that their priority in this placement was to consolidate their clinical skills. This can clearly also impact the achievement of sign-off proficiency by students during the final practice placement, which is an NMC requirement for them to register their qualification with the NMC.

It is useful to note, however, that the notion of learning pathways is found in at least another two contexts. One of these is the arena of adult education in which individuals who have missed education opportunities during compulsory education years are enabled to learn through NVQ routes, and so on (e.g. McGivney, 2003). The notion of learning pathways also belongs to neurophysiology when new learning can be identified along neuronal paths (e.g. Brown et al., 1999). However, this discussion indicates that integrated care pathways lend themselves to 'inter-professional learning pathways' by virtue of the range of healthcare professionals who might be involved in the patient's journey.

## Guidelines, policies and standards for practice placements

In *Helping Students Get the Best from Their Practice Placements*, the Royal College of Nursing (RCN) (2002) specifies the responsibilities of various stakeholders, that is, those of the student, the HEI, service providers, personal tutors and mentors, for ensuring effective learning during placements. The responsibilities of the student encompass those before, during and after the placement. The student's responsibilities before the placement include:

- Reading the student handbooks related to the specific programme of study, including the assessment of practice that must be achieved.
- Recognising the purpose of the practice placement experience which is to learn nursing or midwifery care.
- Contacting the placement.
- Acting professionally with regard to punctuality and attitude, and dress according to uniform policy.

During the placement, the student's responsibility includes being proactive in seeking out learning experiences. After the placement, the student has a responsibility to take stock of their achievements, evaluate the placement itself, ensure all practice placement documentation is completed by due dates and reflect on the experience after completing the placement.

For mentors, the RCN publication states that good mentoring depends on well-planned learning opportunities and the provision of support and coaching for students. It lists and explains several actions that the mentor should take to fulfil their responsibility, which include:

- Contributing to a supportive learning environment and quality learning outcomes for students.
- Being approachable, supportive and aware of how students learn best.
- Having knowledge and information of the student's programme of study and practice assessment tools.

In a subsequent publication that constitutes guidance for mentors, the RCN (2007) addresses how to mentor. This includes mentors helping students get the best from practice placements, including students with special needs, areas of accountability of mentors and support for mentors.

The underlying principles of the DH (2001b) guidance document *Placements in Focus* includes the need for a dynamic and proactive approach to the organisation, provision and assessment of practice experience. It indicates that HEIs and service providers have to think creatively about how to plan and provide practice placements that meet the needs of the NHS, the wider healthcare sector and developments related to public health. Planning and provision should both take into account, and value, ideas and suggestions from students and draw on the experience and knowledge of other stakeholders. The guidance is intended to constitute a model of good practice. It focuses on four key aspects of practice placements, namely:

1  Providing practice placements.
2  Practice learning environment.
3  Student support.
4  Assessment of practice.

For the practice learning environment, the DH (2001b) indicates, for instance, that:

- The practice area should have a stated philosophy of care that is reflected in practice and in the curriculum aims.
- Care provision should be founded on relevant research- and evidence-based findings where available.
- Students should gain, where possible, experience as part of a multi-professional team.

- A learning resources area with relevant materials should be available for learning activities in the practice environment.
- Student feedback should be actively sought.

It also identifies how each component will be achieved by, for instance, placement providers, HEIs and students. Another authoritative body that provides guidelines on placement learning as a 'code of practice' for quality assurance is the Quality Assurance Agency (QAA) (2007). Mulholland et al. make further recommendations under the *Making Practice-based Learning Work* (2006) project.

# Work-Based Learning

In addition to statutory (e.g. DH, 1999) and job-related reasons for the mentor function, other reasons and perspectives emanate from research findings and expert opinions. Kramer's (1974) research on newly qualified nurses constitutes one perspective that was mentioned in Chapter 1; another is the social learning theory advocated by Bandura (1997). Since this theory is firmly based on learning from other people, and this is how healthcare skills are usually learnt, the concept of work-based learning gradually evolved in recognition that learners learn knowledge and skills from competent professionals during care delivery. This section therefore examines what work-based learning (WBL is also referred to as 'practice-based learning') is, its features, research on the concept and related issues.

## What is work-based learning?

Over a decade ago, Guile and Young (1996) identified WBL as an innovative concept that firmly emphasised the importance of the workplace in competence development. They put forward a then relatively controversial idea that learning which does not take place in academic contexts was as important as learning within higher education, and the notion that all work-based learning is valid and creditworthy. Its value could therefore be assessed on the basis of how far it is integrated and possibly accredited within academic programmes, which Chalmers et al. (2001) and Hargreaves (1996) report as achievable. Credit rating of practice modules in the nursing curriculum is now commonplace.

Dewar and Walker (1999) suggest that WBL is primarily concerned with the process of learning and with encouraging the individual to be explicit about how and what they learn so that this experiential learning can also be assessed. Flanagan et al. (2000) note that WBL is the bringing together of self-knowledge, expertise at work and formal knowledge. It takes a structured and learner-managed approach to maximising opportunities for learning and professional development. Barr (2003) defined work-based learning as learning that takes place at work or learning that takes place away from work with the objective of improving performance at work. The definitions of WBL therefore emphasise the link between learning and work role, and interrelate:

1   Structured learning in the workplace.
2   On-the-job training opportunities.
3   Identifying relevant off-job learning situations.
4   Quantifying and credit-rating learning in practice settings.

## Issues and success stories related to WBL

Guile and Young (1996) also suggested that one of the issues with WBL is the limitation of the concept 'competence', which is what is learnt in WBL but which tends to incorporate behaviourist assumptions, with the tendency to relegate competency to reductionist descriptions of skill performance. They conclude that learning a competency should not be limited to 'know-how'; it should explicitly evidence the individual's understanding of the underpinning knowledge. The second issue involves comparability and equivalence between academic and work-based learning. As WBL is still a developing concept, a SWOT analysis of the concept can be undertaken to explore its strengths and problematic areas.

## Activity 4.6   Critical analysis of WBL

Based on the above discussion, do a SWOT analysis of WBL and make notes on what you feel are the likely strengths, weaknesses, opportunities and threats related to WBL in your practice setting.

In response to Activity 4.6, for strengths of WBL you might have mentioned that students get to learn hands-on clinical skills in the actual practice setting (as opposed to learning them in the more artificial surroundings of university skills laboratories), and observe their beneficial impact on the patient's or service user's health; for weaknesses 'lack of time to reflect'; for opportunities 'the chance to learn specialist skills'; and for threats you might have mentioned safety issues.

Following SWOT analysis, action can be taken to rectify or avoid weaknesses and threats. To resolve some of these dilemmas, Guile and Young (1996) recommended the use of the 'connective model', that is, the combination and interdependence of 'theoretical learning' and 'practical learning'. Theoretical learning provides concepts for analysing elements of practice, while practical learning constitutes workplace experience as a key source of competent development. Effective partnership between universities and healthcare providers is a necessary requirement for this to occur.

Components of a SWOT analysis of WBL are presented in Table 4.1, and you might wish to make notes on probable actions against each item.

**TABLE 4.1**  SWOT analysis of WBL and probable actions

| SWOT analysis | Probable actions |
|---|---|
| *Strengths*<br>Learn hands-on practice skills<br>Instil/build confidence<br>Involves multidisciplinary team functioning<br>Can visit other practice areas<br>Is grounded in the real world, i.e. realistic within resource constraints<br>Is more patient-centred<br>Learners question rationales/effects of interventions<br>Is dynamic, i.e. when the patient's condition changes, treatment is adapted | |
| *Weaknesses*<br>Lack of time to reflect<br>Work within resource constraints, therefore minimum/safe standards rather than optimum/expert<br>Learner might not appreciate depth of theoretical knowledge required in e.g. blood pressure recording and monitoring<br>In mental health, may not be able to get out of a patient interaction situation | |
| *Opportunities*<br>Learn specialist skills<br>To practise clinical skills<br>Explore if would like to work there<br>Accredit practice-based learning with higher education credit points<br>To develop clinical practice, i.e. new ideas where there are problems, challenges<br>Multi-professional learning<br>Identify learning needs | |
| *Threats*<br>Safety issues<br>Relatives can oppose learners being involved<br>Insufficient theoretical knowledge<br>Reflection-in-action only, not reflection-on-action<br>Less need for universities<br>Big responsibility on the learner – they might have neither the motivation nor the capacity to know what to learn and how | |

Research studies and evaluation of WBL report variable findings. Some report how WBL programmes have been successfully implemented, while others highlight issues. For instance, Rattray et al. (2006) report on the evaluation of a critical care module that incorporated WBL and resulted in various benefits such as module credibility through its clinical focus. Waddington and Marsh (1998) explored work-based shared learning with a multi-grade, multi-skilled group of qualified nurses and healthcare assistants, and found that the perceived benefits included increased professional awareness of issues relating to standards and quality of care with enhanced communication and morale within the team.

On the other hand, Mallik and McGowan (2007) report on a multi-professional 'developmental project' on WBL which indicates that an inadequate supply of mentors results in inconsistency in the amount of mentoring students receive. Dewar and Walker (1999) report on an evaluation of WBL within a post-registration community health nursing degree programme which revealed a gap between the educational philosophy of WBL and the way in which it was delivered within the department concerned.

Rigorous quantitative studies are as yet in short supply, but Wilson et al. (1998), for instance, report on a qualitative study of continuing professional development within a selection of healthcare organisations, which indicates that a number of interrelated factors contribute to WBL. These factors include: (a) the involvement of senior staff whose visions of learning make them role models for novice practitioners; (b) organisational structures and sufficient resources that support effective teamwork; (c) prompt feedback on performance to enable further learning to take place. The main conclusions indicate that the concept of a learning organisation was not readily recognised within healthcare, although some of their components were.

Ward and McCormack (2000) suggest that the development of a learning culture is becoming a dominant theme in the strategic plans of healthcare organisations. This is arising through a drive to improve standards of practice, bridging the perceived theory–practice gap and creating the means of integrating learning with practice. There have been many initiatives to create such a change, including CPD, reflective practice, clinical supervision and WBL.

Spouse (2001b) notes that successful WBL requires an organisational environment that supports learning through investment in staff, with staffing structures in organisations and trusts that free people up to work and learn collaboratively in a climate of trust, where investigations and speculations are fostered, and where time is protected for engaging in discussions about practice.

## Becoming a learning organisation

In line with Wilson et al.'s (1998) and Ward and McCormack's (2000) suggestions that organisational factors have a major influence on learning, the term 'practice learning environment' is increasingly being seen as connected to the concept 'learning organisation'. This concept is part of a trio of notions that include lifelong learning and learning society. It evolved with the development of various non-healthcare organisations such as banks, supermarkets, and so on, as learning organisations on the basis that they all learn from customer feedback and actively engage in ongoing staff training.

Watkins and Marsick (1992: 118) note that learning organisations are 'characterised by total employee involvement in a process of collaboratively initiated, collaboratively conducted, collectively accountable change direction towards shared values and principles'. The concept of a learning organisation is consistently becoming a feature of healthcare settings, as lifelong learning is not merely 'keeping up to date', but encompasses a flexible and enquiring approach to the development of a culture of learning as an important part of the work setting.

As for learning society, de la Harpe and Radloff (2000: 169) note this comprises a society in which 'every person has the opportunity to be educated to the level of achievement of which they are truly capable'. Healthcare trusts and smaller healthcare units can be viewed as learning organisations if they manifest such attributes or features as:

- Having a clearly articulated mission statement that puts patient or service users at the centre of all their activities.
- Effective communication throughout the organisation – top-down and bottom-up communication, verbally, by holding regular meetings, information via e-mails, etc.
- Key stakeholders and practitioners at all levels and range of the organisation are involved in its development, including multi-disciplinary groups, voluntary groups, etc.
- A firm professional development strategy is in place for all employees, which is a dimension of performance reviews and incorporates personal development plans (PDP).
- Clinical supervision accessible for practitioners for peer support, and for developing PDPs.
- Recognition provided that learning takes place in the workplace, and incorporates WBL, IPL and provision of mentorship.
- Translation of rhetoric into action, for example named nurse, team midwifery, acting on audit findings.
- Commitment to engagement in reflective practice.

## Issues Related to Practice Placements

One of the issues related to pre-registration nursing students is their supernumerary status accompanied by a relatively small bursary, as indicated at the end of Chapter 2. The latter is a reason for a number of students holding down part-time jobs. This, along with some students having a family to support, may result in their learning being compromised to some extent.

Consequently, the student is likely to need extra structured support while on practice placement. Link tutors can provide this support, which doesn't necessarily require their physical presence.

A study by Young et al. (2010) evaluated the use of short message service (SMS) texting between university staff and students as an additional means of support for healthcare students (including Nursing, Radiography and Occupational Therapy students) during practice placements. They found that texting can improve students' access to additional support when needed during practice placements.

One of the reasons for various guidelines on practice placements being issued by the RCN, the QAA, the DH (e.g. DH, 2001b) and others at the turn of the last century is the findings of research by Phillips et al. (2000), which documents various worrying weaknesses with prevailing mentoring processes. As noted in Chapter 1, this study highlights several issues or problems experienced by both mentors and students which resulted in a redefinition of roles and a change in educational preparation programmes for mentors.

Another reason is the increase in the number of students due to the shortage of qualified nurses. This means that more learners were to be mentored by fewer RNs. This also coincides with other research findings that some mentors were failing to fail students (discussed in Chapter 7) who were not competent, and that some newly qualified RNs were not 'fit for practice', that is, not clinically competent.

On the other hand, the heightened awareness of evidence-based practice means that students are more inquisitive about reasons for each step within clinical interventions. However, for various day-to-day reasons, some procedures are not performed exactly as the procedures' manual states, and consequently the so-called theory and practice gap at times surfaces. From qualified healthcare professionals' and their managers' viewpoint these still constitute competent practice because procedures are adapted in accordance with resource availability and patient circumstances. For instance, if the moving and handling procedure or guidelines state that a hoist should be used to help a patient above a certain weight, but a hoist is not immediately available, then the RN could use alternative measures. The reason for this might not be immediately obvious to the student, and at times students refuse to participate in procedures that are not being performed precisely according to guidelines. They should be exploring how to adapt theories to practice instead.

## Chapter Summary

As with other components in this book, creating and maintaining an effective practice learning environment is also identified as a key component of the mentor role. This chapter has focused on the different ways in which practice settings can be effective as learning environments, and has therefore explored:

- Student's perspectives on practice placements such as their hopes and expectations, a ward orientation or induction programme, advanced preparation of learners, and ensuring that course practice competencies are achieved.
- Research on practice learning environments, which underpins the development of the tool for annual educational audits of practice placement areas; learning resources (human and material) including inter-professional learning, and learning pathways; role models for learners in the practice setting.
- The part played by national guidelines, standards and current policy documents on practice placements.
- What is work-based learning? How work-based learning is perceived and implemented, and an analysis of issues and success stories related to work-based learning, and successful implementation thereof.
- Some of the main issues related to practice placements for students.

## Further Optional Reading

For practical and contemporary guidance on how to enhance the quality of practice placements for healthcare trust-based professionals, including AHPs, that builds on previous work and on evidence about students' experience of practice, and prepared collaboratively by a number of statutory and professional bodies and the Department of Health, as well as a complementary element of quality assurance of NHS funded health professional education programmes, see:

- *Placement in Focus: Guidance for Education in Practice for Healthcare Professions* (DH, 2001b). Available at: www.dh.gov.uk/en/Publicationsandstatistics/Publications/PublicationsPolicyAndGuidance/DH_4009511. Accessed 10 May 2010.

For the QAA's stance on effective learning during practice placements, see:

- Quality Assurance Agency for Higher Education (2007) *Code of Practice for the Assurance of Academic Quality and Standards in Higher Education. Section 9: Work-based and Placement Learning.* Available at: www.qaa.ac.uk/academicinfrastructure/codeofpractice/section9/placementlearning.pdf. Accessed 12 July 2010.

# 5
# Effective Practice and Clinical Practice Development

## Introduction

The key dimensions of being a mentor in healthcare professions incorporate practising one's craft to the highest standard. This in turn implies being conscious of the quality and effectiveness of one's practice, continuously ascertaining the evidence base of all clinical interventions, and of the various factors that influence effective delivery of patients and service users' care and treatment. Awareness of standards of practice involves being open-minded with regards to novel methods of clinical interventions, of developments in one's own specialist field of practice.

The NMC's (2008a: 56–7) standards document indicates under the domain 'Context of practice', that the mentor must 'Support learning within a context of practice that reflects healthcare and educational policies, managing change to ensure that particular professional needs are met within a learning environment that also supports practice development'. Under 'Evidence-based practice', the NMC indicates that the mentor must 'Apply evidence-based practice to their own work and contribute to the further development of such knowledge, and practice evidence base'. The outcomes for these domains are:

- Context of practice
  - contribute to the development of an environment in which effective practice is fostered, implemented, evaluated and disseminated
  - set and maintain professional boundaries that are sufficiently flexible for providing inter-professional care

- initiate and respond to practice developments to ensure safe and effective care is achieved and an effective learning environment is maintained

- Evidence-based
  - identify and apply research and evidence-based practice to practice in their area of practice
  - contribute to strategies to increase or review the evidence base used to support practice
  - support students in applying an evidence base to their own practice

The concepts inherent within these requirements and outcomes are addressed in this chapter, which are predominantly key components of effective and evidence-based practice (EBP), practice development and the management of change.

## Chapter outcomes

On completion of this chapter, you should be able to:

1  Explain why effective care and clinical practice development are key components of the RN's/RM's mentor role.
2  Ascertain what the concepts 'effective care' and 'clinical practice development' signify, and identify the inherent components that they encompass.
3  Ascertain and analyse what is EBP and how comprehensively the mentor engages in this.
4  Evaluate how mentors can engage in, develop and disseminate effective practice.
5  Critically evaluate how the mentor can be involved in the effective implementation of research findings, and the management of change.

## Effective Practice

'Effective clinical practice' is a concept that is closely related to quality assurance and is part of the quality agendas in the UK, such as clinical governance, and the work of the NHS Institute for Innovation and Improvement (NHS III) (2010) whose work includes projects and rigorous testing of new ways of providing care in such areas as long-term conditions, primary care, end of life care and mental health services. Effective care (NMC, 2008a) is a concept that is an integral component of EBP, and is also closely related to the terms *clinical effectiveness* and *patient outcomes*.

'Clinical effectiveness' refers to the extent to which specific clinical interventions, when deployed in the field for a particular patient or population, do what they are intended to do, that is, restore and improve health and secure the greatest possible health gain from the available resources (DH, 1996). The

RCN (1996) took this definition a stage further, indicating that clinical effectiveness is about applying the best available knowledge, which is derived from
research, clinical expertise and patient preferences, to achieve optimum outcomes for patients. It emphasises maximum restoration of health, which is
undertaken at the highest standard achievable. The three stages for achieving
clinical effectiveness are (DH, 1996):

- Obtaining evidence – from research published in journals, databases, clinical guidelines
  and so on.
- Implementing the evidence.
- Evaluating the impact of the changed practice and readjusting practice as necessary,
  usually through clinical audit and patient feedback.

The word *effective* is an adjective, which according to the dictionary (Brown,
2002: 794) means 'capable of producing results or a condition, and having the
function of accomplishing or executing'. It can be used interchangeably with
'efficacious' and 'productive'. Related to the mentor role, the word effective
therefore implies that the qualified healthcare professional accomplishes
the goals in their patients' or service users' plans of care and treatment (or care
pathways), as intended. So, effective care, clinical effectiveness and practice
development all aim to monitor and improve the standards and quality of
healthcare delivery.

The three stages of achieving clinical effectiveness incorporate EBP and
practice development, which are examined in detail shortly. Achieving the
goals of care and treatment also belongs to the arena of *patient outcomes*. This
term has been explored for several years, and is defined according to the
research it is connected with, as documented by the RCN (2004). However,
despite the logic in ascertaining patient outcomes, there is a lack of consensus with regard to how patient outcomes are gauged, and therefore it remains
in the background as an essential notion warranting further research and
refinement.

The remainder of this chapter focuses on EBP and practice development
as components of mentors' roles and then management of change.

## Evidence-Based Practice

One of the crucial components of effective practice and clinical governance
is EBP, a concept that has been gradually adopted in all areas of healthcare. As
indicated at the beginning of the chapter, besides being one of the NMC's
(2008a) competences for mentors, EBP is also usually a component of the
codes of practice of healthcare professionals. So what is EBP?

## What is evidence-based practice?

Evidence-based practice is closely associated with evidence-based medicine, for which Dr Archie Cochrane is renowned for being one of its principal initiators (Clarke, 1999). Sackett et al. (2000) are also well known for being advocates of EBP, and according to them EBP is the conscientious, explicit and judicious use of current best evidence in making decisions about the care of individual patients.

The key reasons for the adoption of EBP in healthcare is the move towards ensuring patient involvement in their care and treatment, the rise of consumerism and the shift from traditional or routine procedures to more objective scientific working (Dale, 2006).

Another term related to EBP is 'evidence-based healthcare' (EBHC), and it has permeated various areas of organisational function in the form of evidence-based nursing, evidence-based management and evidence-based education. EBHC is defined by Gray (2001: 9) as 'a discipline centred upon evidence-based decision-making about groups of patients, or populations, which can manifest itself as evidence-based policy-making, purchasing or management'. Although they overlap substantially, EBHC can be distinguished from EBP in that the former tends to refer to groups of patients, while the latter can refer to single clinical interventions. According to Gray, there are five key elements of EBP, namely:

1   Decisions are based on best evidence.
2   The nature and source of evidence are determined by the problem.
3   Best evidence integrates research and personal experience.
4   Evidence is translated into action that affects patients/service users.
5   These actions are continually appraised.

### Best evidence

EBP therefore refers to the use of 'best evidence' and is based on national and international standards. How do we know that the way we provide care and treatment in our workplace is based on the 'best evidence' currently available?

**Think Point 5.1**

Research evidence is available from national computer databases. However, Gray (2001) indicates that although the best evidence of effectiveness of particular clinical interventions comes from well-designed research, other evidence of best practice, referred to as 'best evidence available', needs to be considered seriously. There are several likely sources of best evidence of good practice, including:

- policy directives (from the Department of Health);
- specialist and research conferences;
- professional journal articles;
- overview of evidence on specific topics on computer databases;
- textbooks;
- suppliers' information;
- unpublished research;
- suggestions from patients with a particular health problem;
- colleagues and peer contact – uni- or inter-disciplinary professionals;
- clinical guidelines;
- the patient/service user/their family;
- personal intuition;
- trial and error;
- personal experience.

## How is EBP achieved?

There are various ways in which EBP can be achieved. Healthcare professionals can search for evidence of the effect of particular clinical interventions and best evidence on computer databases such as the Cochrane library, MEDLINE or Cumulative Index to Nursing and Allied Health Literature (CINAHL), or they can do a manual search of targeted literature.

There are various organisations that store and provide systematically reviewed (or critically appraised, or meta-analysed) research on different healthcare topics. The Cochrane systematic reviews library (available at www.cochrane.de/default.html), which stores research evidence that has been appraised or systematically reviewed, is one of them. Sleep and Clark (1999: 306–7) define a systematic review as 'a rigorous and exhaustive process for searching and appraising both published and unpublished literature on a specific aspect of healthcare … they adhere to strict scientific design in order to make them more comprehensive, to minimise the chance of bias, and so ensure their reliability'.

The strengths of the assembled research literature can be classified as a hierarchy of levels or grades of evidence, in order of validity and significance. Hemingway and Brereton (2009: 7), for instance, classify 'Hierarchies of evidence' at five levels of evidence (and sub-levels), as follows:

- Level 1a   Systematic review (with homogeneity) of randomised controlled trials (RCTs)
- Level 1b   Individual RCT (with narrow confidence interval)
- Level 1c   All-or-none studies
- Level 2a   Systematic review (with homogeneity) of cohort studies
- Level 2b   Individual cohort study (including low-quality RCT; e.g. < 80% follow-up)
- Level 2c   'Outcomes' research; ecological studies
- Level 3a   Systematic reviews (with homogeneity) of case-control studies

- Level 3b   Individual case-control study
- Level 4    Case series (and poor quality cohort and case-control studies)
- Level 5    Expert opinion without explicit critical appraisal, or based on physiology, bench research or 'first principles'

Other organisations categorise evidence differently but they are essentially similar. Evans (2003) explored various such classifications and concluded that the appraisal of evidence should also include assessing the evidence's effectiveness, appropriateness and feasibility. Nonetheless, Sackett et al. (1996), Rolfe (1999) and others indicate strongly that RCTs must not be treated as 'gold standards'. Thompson (1998) and others indicate that EBP should take personal experience, intuition and patients' reports into account. The benefits of EBP are that healthcare professionals can (Kopp, 2001):

- Inform or advise patients more accurately.
- Make better use of limited resources.
- Instigate appropriate and up-to-date interventions.
- Measure practice against appropriate guidelines or standards.
- Provide a more informed decision-making process to previously untreatable or more expensive treatments.

However, there can be barriers to the implementation of EBP. These barriers are similar to those that present as obstacles to implementation of research findings and are examined shortly. Kopp (2001) suggests that such barriers include a lack of awareness of evidence, and of self-confidence, peer support or resources. Furthermore, Sackett et al. (1996: 71) suggest that 'practice risks becoming tyrannised by evidence ... [but] without available evidence, practice risks becoming rapidly out of date to the detriment of patients'.

The difference between research-based practice and EBP is that research-based practice of clinical interventions usually only allows consideration of findings of quantitative research, while EBP also considers descriptive or qualitative studies, professional experiences, intuition (Benner, 2001) and tacit knowledge (when we know more than we can evidence or tell) (Polanyi, 1958).

The York University NHS Centre for Reviews and Dissemination is another resource centre for EBP. There is also the quarterly journal *Evidence-based Nursing*. The Health Technology Assessment programme (DH, 2010c) is a government-funded venture that appraises research information, including costs and effectiveness, and is made available to NHS workers. Typical headings for appraisal of a research study are:

- How clear and specific is the research question?
- Was the research funded by a particular organisation and, if so, does the researcher hold any allegiance to them?

- Is the research design the most appropriate to answer the research question?
- Are the sampling strategies the most appropriate?
- Precisely what was measured?
- Precise details and relevance of how the data was collected.
- How researcher effects and other intervening variables were controlled.
- Was the framework or method used for analysing the data the most appropriate?
- Are the statistical tests used appropriate and accurately documented?
- Are the conclusions drawn logically argued and is the generalisability statement justifiable?
- To what extent is the study relevant to clinical practice in the particular practice setting?
- Does the dissemination of the study indicate frameworks for implementation, including resources required such as costs?

Much more detailed appraisal considerations are pretty well publicised, and guidelines for systematic reviews are provided, for example, by Gopee (2010). It is in the interest of the implementer of a particular component of EBP to examine closely and carefully the appraisal or systematic review already conducted by established organisations, who in fact are also likely to have accessed and appraised the original study report.

## The mentor's role in identifying, disseminating and applying research findings

Identifying existing research on particular healthcare topic areas or components of clinical practice has become increasingly easier with the wide availability of electronic databases such as the Cochrane library and MEDLINE. However, the actual dissemination of research findings is often not as effectively achieved. Whether it is the findings of the healthcare professional's own research or those of studies encountered at conferences or on courses, the ultimate stages of research studies entail critiquing the study or studies, systematic dissemination and implementation of the findings.

McKenna (1995) noted that just getting the findings or a new idea published in a professional journal amounts to researchers simply reporting their findings, making recommendations and opting out, in the hope that someone will implement their recommendations. Dissemination by this single avenue therefore has limited impact. Scullion (2002) suggests that dissemination is a vital yet complex process that aims to ensure that key messages are conveyed to specific groups via a wide range of methods such that it results in impact, reaction and preferably implementation. Scullion suggests that the range of methods for effective dissemination include:

- journal articles/editorials/short reports;
- feedback to research subjects;
- in-person support mechanisms;

- journal clubs;
- seminars;
- conference presentations;
- poster presentations;
- publishing as books/chapters;
- inclusion in curriculum;
- newsletters;
- designing educational materials.

Scullion (2002) suggests that the main barriers to the dissemination process are: poor reading habits of nurses resulting in them being unaware of research findings, lack of time, lack of knowledge, negative attitudes towards research and information overload. However, to disseminate new research-based or innovative practice, Price (2010) provides guidance on specific strategies that can be used, such as planning for the specific audience, identifying objectives for the session, and use of artefacts (e.g. plastic models of body parts, etc.).

Furthermore, even with effective dissemination, there can be obstacles to the implementation of research findings. Decades ago, Hunt (1981) identified the 'major obstacles to applying research in practice' as nurses not knowing about research findings, not understanding them, not believing in them, not knowing how to use them and not being allowed to use them. Education curricula for healthcare professionals have over the years ensured inclusion of research modules, but some years after her initial study, Hunt (1997) again explored the barriers to research implementation faced by both nurse managers and clinicians and found that these include:

- Lack of critical appraisal and research skills.
- Lack of time to undertake research.
- Not having access to the right resources.
- An organisational and managerial ethos and culture expecting instant answers.
- Lack of power and financial control to make things happen.
- Lack of valid research on any one topic, or of user-friendly reviews and guidelines.

## Barriers to implementing research findings

Consider Hunt's (1997) findings for yourself, or discuss with an appropriate colleague, how far the findings are still prevalent in the context of present-day healthcare settings, both in general and in your own practice setting.

Think
Point 5.2

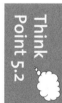

McCaughan et al. (2002) explored acute care nurses' perceptions of barriers to using research information in clinical decision-making, and identified them as:

- Problems in interpreting and using research, as they are seen as too complex, 'academic' and overly statistical.
- Nurses who feel confident with research-based information perceive a lack of organisational support.
- Researchers and findings lack clinical credibility and fail to offer sufficient clinical direction.
- Some nurses lack the skills and motivation to use research themselves.
- Participants like research messages passed on to them by a third party rather than becoming directly involved themselves.
- Rejection of research knowledge is not a barrier to its application, but the presentation and management of research knowledge in the workplace represent significant challenges for clinicians, policy-makers and the research community.

---

## Activity 5.1    Barriers to implementation of research findings

Re-read the barriers to implementation of research findings identified by Hunt and McCaughan in the previous bulleted lists, and consider what you see as barriers in your workplace, at ward or trust level, and make some notes.

---

Implementing changes to practice is examined later in this chapter. Palfreyman et al. (2003) explored nurses' and physiotherapists' sources of knowledge and perceived barriers to EBP, and found that although both parties access a wide variety of sources of knowledge, both professions have problems overcoming the barrier of time. Furthermore, nurses are more likely to use policy and procedure manuals, but rate themselves as having poor EBP skills. Hunt (1997), however, suggests that these issues can be resolved by:

- Making research available and accessible by development programmes.
- Providing research advice and support.
- Providing nurses with the appropriate skills.
- Changing attitudes.

On the other hand, Scullion (2002) notes that current commitment to research and EBP will have limited impact on patient care unless a similar commitment to dissemination and implementation is established at both corporate and individual levels. Rycroft–Malone et al. (2002) note that successful implementation of evidence into practice is a function of three elements, namely the nature of the evidence, the context in which the change is to take place and the way the process is managed. They suggest a framework based on these elements for both implementation of novel practices and subsequent evaluation.

In the mentoring role, research–based practice is an inherent component. EBP can be a permanent feature, and 'where's the evidence?' sounds like a confrontational question. The healthcare trust's clinical procedure and guidelines, however, almost always include the evidence base for practice. Consider the following scenario which involves mentoring a student midwife.

## 📁 Case Study – Mentoring a student midwife

Sarah is the mentor to first-year student midwife, Helen. A 'triad'* assessment is being conducted with Helen by Sarah and Geraldine, the link tutor. The topic chosen is examination of the newborn.

Helen states that she is very nervous. She provides a full clinical picture of the woman and the baby in whose care she has been involved. Having confirmed the woman's consent, she then concentrates on the examination, which she performs in a professional manner. There is, however, little communication with the mother. Helen has to be reminded of the need to complete the relevant documentation. Her hand is shaking as she writes.

Helen then produces and discusses an article regarding examinations of the healthy neonate. She needs some prompting when asked about the NMC's *Midwives Rules and Standards* and what she would do if she identified a deviation from the norm. When asked about her assessment of her performance, Helen is very self-critical, and feels that she did not do very well.

What are the key issues in this assessment situation? What are the ways in which the evidence base of Helen's performance influenced her performance, and what are the questions that Sarah and Geraldine might want to ask?

*triad* refers to a tri-partite assessment of competencies in the practice setting that includes the assessee, their mentor and a midwife lecturer.

You do not have to be a midwife to ask relevant questions related to EBP and this case study, and a number of issues surface when this scenario is put to group discussions. In the context of the discussions in this chapter, all parties will question the strengths of the evidence that Helen seemed to have used during the procedure. They can be explored in the context of levels or grades of evidence available in relation to 'examination of the newborn'.

# Clinical Practice Development

The two concepts of clinical effectiveness and EBP both imply changing the ways in which care and treatment are delivered if it benefits the patient or service user. Such changes are referred to as 'clinical practice development', which is the focus of the next section of this chapter. Clinical practice development is a key component of the NMC (2008a) competences for mentors. This section explores what clinical practice development is, the different reasons for practice development and how these developments are managed, which links up to the next section of this chapter on management of change.

## What is clinical practice development?

Clinical practice development implies changing the way particular care and treatment interventions are performed for the benefit of patients or service users. It has to do with improving and enhancing clinical practice where there is scope to do so. It refers to hands-on patient care interventions, that is patient contact. Which developments in clinical practice are currently happening in your particular area of practice? What changes can be made or have been made recently to the specific care and treatments carried out in your practice setting?

---

### Activity 5.2   Clinical practice development

Reflect on how care is currently delivered in your workplace and explore whether any aspect of hands-on patient care has changed recently – in the last few months, or in the last year or two?
   Next, identify an aspect of practice in your work setting that requires or could benefit from change, either in clinical care, patient teaching or organisation of care. State two examples of such potential changes.

---

So, changes can be made in different components or dimensions of the healthcare professional's role. The mentor can influence the nature and direction of these changes. Examples of changes in hands–on clinical practice include:

- no-lift policy;
- use of patient-controlled analgesia;
- nurse-led specialist clinics;
- cognitive-behavioural therapy;
- nurse prescribing;

- using tympanic thermometers rather than glass thermometers;
- cardiac output studies in intensive care units;
- bedside handover;
- a red jug of water next to a patient who is at risk of dehydration.

## Examples of changes in organisation or management of care include:

- introducing a new shift system;
- integrated care pathways;
- team midwifery;
- outreach work;
- a quality assurance programme (e.g. patient satisfaction surveys);
- modern matron role in aspects of care (e.g. who does what to ensure hospital cleanliness);
- allowing parents to be present in the anaesthetic room;
- clinical supervision for peer support and CPD;
- a mechanism for reporting to colleagues from conferences and workshops.

## Examples of changes in patient teaching include:

- health 'MOTs' conducted by practice nurses, SCPHNs;
- school nurses' advice to teenagers on sexual activity;
- teaching self-relaxation;
- teaching dietary control to a newly diagnosed diabetic;
- advising older people on how to avoid hypothermia.

You could think of various instances of changes in teaching students and other learners, such as medical students, healthcare assistants, preceptees and inductees.

Practice development is defined by the RCN (2006: 1) as 'an approach that helps you, your team and organisation to provide care that patients feel is right for them'. This is a very brief definition. A more helpful definition is provided by McCormack et al. (1999: 256), which states that:

> Practice development is a continuous process of improvement towards increased effectiveness in person-centred care, through the enabling of nurses and healthcare teams to transform the culture and context of care. It is enabled and supported by facilitators committed to a systematic, rigorous and continuous process of emanci-patory change.

According to Bryar and Griffiths (2003), practice development is taken to mean a broad range of innovations that are initiated to improve practice and the services in which that practice takes place. The term *innovation* differs from practice development in certain respects, especially in that the former refers to implementing something new and unprecedented. The dictionary (Brown, 2002: 1381) defines 'innovate' as introducing 'something for the first time, a new product, practice or method', and 'to make a change to something established'. Both activities refer to something developed necessarily in response to patient care needs, but development refers to a gradual progressive change and advancement. Innovation implies implementing a relatively radical new practice. Change as a concept, however, can mean substituting something with something new, a development, or reverting to an older (but effective) practice.

Although nursing practice has been developing consistently over the years, one of the key stages in this is marked by the establishment of Nursing Development Units in the 1980s, which were practice settings where appropriate changes in practice were implemented and empirically evaluated.

## Why clinical practice development?

One of the primary reasons that practice development is a mentoring role is that mentors are role models for their learners (Darling, 1984; NMC, 2008a). This reason complements the role or characteristic of the mentor as a standard-prodder, identified by Darling (1984), which implies that they should always be reflecting on whether their clinical interventions are of the highest standard known, with a view to making them even more effective.

The two NMC domains clearly indicate that the mentor must continually question the evidence base and effectiveness of the care they deliver. However, clinical practice is only one of the components of the RN's role that can be developed, others being their education and management roles. Another categorisation of healthcare professionals' roles, each of which can be further developed, is by the Department of Health (2004a) in the *NHS KSF,* which identifies all patient care activities under six 'core dimensions', namely: (i) communication; (ii) personal and people development; (iii) health, safety and security; (iv) service improvement; (v) quality; and (vi) equality and diversity. All categories imply quality assurance, but service improvement in particular relates to making 'changes in own practice and offer suggestions for improving services' (2004a: 70).

Practice development is evolving continually, and Collinson (2000) and Faugier (2005b), for instance, take the concept further and discuss the 'growth' of 'nurse entrepreneurs'. The term *entrepreneur* of course refers to people who engage in novel, unprecedented ventures on a substantial scale, and implies being innovators. Liefer (2005) discusses government policy changes that allow entrepreneurial nurses to pave the way for nurse-led healthcare practices, for instance nurse-led leg ulcer clinics.

The RN's teaching role starts soon after registering as a nurse with the NMC, and they have to be qualified for one year before accessing the mentor preparation course. Therefore, although the mentor needs to monitor the evidence base and effectiveness of their practice, the extent to which they can engage in practice development is variable depending on experience and clinical circumstances. Becoming a nurse entrepreneur is an even longer-term prospect.

Government directives that encourage practice development include *Liberating the Talents* (DH, 2002a), a document that encourages primary care nurses and midwives to develop their practice. It indicates that the Chief Nursing Officer's (DH, 2002b) ten key roles for nurses provides a strategic framework for developing practice, and cites several examples of developments under 'setting up new services'. This is reinforced in various Department of Health documents, including *Modernising Nursing Careers: Setting the Direction* (DH, 2006).

Practice development is also propelled by RNs' expanded roles. Previously known as 'extended roles', 'expanded roles' refer to those clinical interventions that healthcare professionals engage in following relevant post-registration training and assessment.

With the implementation of the *European Working Time Directive* (DH, 2004c) leading to a reduction in doctors' working hours, an increasing range of clinical interventions that were previously doctors' roles are now also performed by other healthcare professionals. These roles afford healthcare professionals greater autonomy and further scope for decision-making, and therefore creativity and consequent practice development, as also noted by the RCN (2005).

A major study by the UKCC (2000) on expanded roles revealed that their impact on practice include:

- Continuity of care being regarded as the most important benefit.
- Practitioners being involved with work in care settings where there is a good skill mix, regular opportunities for CPD, and excellent communications and mutual respect within the healthcare team.
- Professional experience, motivation and use of intuition as well as education and supervision being important practitioners' abilities.

The study also concluded that to support role development, healthcare organisations must provide:

- Adequate training (i.e. CPD).
- Structures which support CPD.
- Management support, sustained by education and training.
- Change that is patient-led rather than management-driven.
- Clear guidelines and protocols.

However, clinical practice development is often triggered by a need for new actions to resolve a health problem. For example, falls amongst older people has presented as an issue for some time, and one of the actions taken by the NHS III (2010) entitled 'High impact actions' addresses this problem, regarding which Ward et al. (2010) report of novel interventions that are being implemented, namely:

- Use of sensor alarms that alert nurses when an 'at risk' patient gets out of bed unaided.
- Identification of a falls team that is led by a matron, whose role includes staff training on the issue/topic area.
- Distraction therapy in dementia.
- A new observation tool to identify the risk of falls.

## Management of clinical practice developments

### Concept analysis of practice development

Garbett and McCormack (2002) undertook a concept analysis of practice development based on an analysis of literature, focus group interviews with practice developers and telephone interviews with practitioners. A conceptual framework derived from the study comprises the purposes, attributes and outcomes of practice development (see Box 5.1).

---

**Box 5.1    Purposes, attributes and outcomes of practice development**

**The purposes of practice development are to:**
- Increase the effectiveness of patient care
- Transform care and the cultures and context within which it takes place

**The attributes of practice development are that it:**
- Requires a systematic and rigorous approach
- Is a continuous process
- Is founded on various types of facilitation

**The consequences of practice development include:**
- For users – improved experiences of care in terms of their sensitivity to the needs of individuals and populations
- For practitioners – increased capacity for thinking creatively and more broadly
- Greater awareness of the impact of organisations on practice

---

Unsworth's (2000) concept analysis of practice development identified wide variations in the way the term is used, and resulted in a tentative list of critical attributes of practice development, which are:

**TABLE 5.1**    A framework for practice development

| Practice development | Structure/approach | Process/deployment | Outcome/results |
|---|---|---|---|
| Individual | Individual performance review/practice development framework | Development of practice development facilitator, or each team member | Active participants Reflective practitioner |
| Unit/Team | ............ | ............ | ............ |
| Organisational | ............ | ............ | ............ |
| Supra-organisational | ............ | ............ | ............ |

*Source*: adapted from Page 2001

- New ways of working which lead to a direct measurable improvement in the care of or service to the client.
- Changes which occur as a response to a specific client need or problem.
- Changes which lead to the development of effective services.
- The maintenance or expansion of business/work.

Titchen (2003) identifies three overarching themes that form the basis for effective practice development, which she refers to as the practice development diamond. The themes are: (a) changing the practice philosophy; (b) the process of change in practice; and (c) investing in professional development. Page (2001) presents a framework of practice development using the Donabedian model, which incorporates developments instigated at individual level, team level, organisational level or at supra-organisational level (see Table 5.1).

The framework is comprehensive and, when all details are completed, it can also be used for ongoing and summative evaluation of the development after it has been implemented.

---

## Activity 5.3    Developing practice

Based on the list of developments generated as a result of Activity 5.2, think of two aspects of practice in your work base that could be developed. Consider and make notes on how the framework presented by Page (2001) can be utilised to change these two aspects of practice.

---

The practice development framework suggested by Page should enable you to take these developments further systematically if you so wish, and maybe within the context of management of change (discussed next in this chapter). The RCN (2006) also has a designated Practice Development Team that provides structured help, advice and support in various ways.

The resources that can help healthcare professionals include the journal *Practice Development in Healthcare*, and national conferences specifically on practice development. Several NHS trusts employ Practice Development Nurses or Facilitators. Some have Practice Development Units that conduct experiments on new modes of practice.

## Managing Change

All healthcare professionals will have encountered changes in the way care and treatment are organised and delivered in various practice settings. It is therefore almost inevitable that mentors will be involved as participants in change, and they are also expected to initiate change as and when appropriate. Therefore, the mentor needs to have knowledge and competence in managing change. It is important to distinguish between the concept of managing change from those of introducing or imposing change; the latter can be effected at short notice, but managing the change implies longer-term, planned and systematic activities. Change is ongoing in healthcare delivery but why do we have changes in healthcare in the first place?

### Why changes in healthcare?

---

### Activity 5.4     Changes in healthcare delivery

Consider the points made about practice development earlier in this chapter, and think of as many reasons as you can for changes that continually occur in healthcare at ward level, hospital level, and in primary and social care settings. Make notes on what you feel are the range of reasons for these changes.

---

Chances are you will have thought of quite a few reasons for changes that you have observed in healthcare. They include government policy directives, such as *The National Service Framework for Long-term Neurological Conditions* (DH, 2008c), or action based on research for increasing productivity in healthcare (Smith and Rudd, 2010), 'high impact actions' (NHS III, 2010), the need to improve practice, and learning from 'near misses' or mistakes. These reasons can be grouped under seven areas, as noted in Box 5.2.

---

## Box 5.2   Reasons for changes in healthcare

- Change in medical technology
- New medical devices and equipments; use of computer networks and easier access to information

- New knowledge
- Research and audit findings; expert guidelines

- Safer and more effective products
- Consumable materials and hardware being superseded by more efficient ones

- The nature of the workforce
- Workers of different age groups, and with domestic responsibilities; changes in qualified: unqualified staff ratio, e.g. healthcare assistants with different skills

- Revised policies and strategies
- Use of devices and strategies to prevent injury to staff, or to avoid 'hospital acquired infections'

- Quality-conscious consumers
- Consumer satisfaction surveys indicating the changes that should be made

- Funding and budgets
- Availability and distribution of scarce resources

---

Consequently, change emanates from various sources, in addition to the mentor's role as evidence-based practitioner and practice developer. In fact, change is an inescapable feature of both organisational and personal life. The many sources of change that you thought of as well as those noted in Box 5.2 can also be grouped under those that are internal to the organisation (e.g. efficiency measures) and those that are external (e.g. legislative changes). However, some reasons can be both internal and external. For instance, if the quality of care is unsatisfactory, then the employees of the organisation will usually be aware of this, and they'll endeavour to rectify it, but the same issue might have been identified through external sources such as Care Quality Commission (CQC) audits.

Seven essential and interrelated factors for successful management of change have been identified by Gopee and Galloway (2009) as the seven-step RAPSIES framework for systematic management of change. The RAPSIES framework entails (in sequence):

1  **Recognition** of the need for change to solve a problem for instance, or to improve an element of practice.
2  **Analysis** of the available options related to the contemplated change, the environment or setting where change will be implemented and the users of the change.

3  **Preparation** for the change, such as identifying a change agent to lead the implementation of the change, education, defining intended outcomes and involving relevant colleagues.
4  **Strategies** for implementing the change.
5  **Implementation** of the change including piloting the change, timing of implementation.
6  **Evaluation** of the impact of the change against the intended outcomes.
7  **Sustaining** the change, i.e. how to ensure the change endures and is mainstreamed.

The change could succeed or fail, depending on the effectiveness of each of the seven steps in the framework. For example, if integrated care pathways (discussed in Chapter 4) are to be implemented, then have each of the seven steps been managed effectively? Further details on each of these steps are as follows.

## Recognition of the need for change

The key attributes that are necessary in the innovation or change if it is to be implemented successfully, are:

- *Relative advantage* – the change must show that it has relative advantage over the status quo.
- *Compatibility* – the proposed change must be compatible with existing beliefs and values of the group at philosophical as well as at pragmatic levels.
- *Communicability* – the ease with which the change can be understood.
- *Simplicity* – the ease or difficulty in the use of the innovation.
- *Trialability* – possibility of piloting the innovation, to identify and resolve unanticipated issues.
- *Observability* – the change must be observable.
- *Relevance* – the degree to which the change is relevant for the particular practice setting.

Therefore, if there is recognition of the need for change to integrated care pathways, then the questions need to be asked whether it is to the advantage of patients and service users compared to how care and treatment are currently delivered; whether the concept is compatible with the healthcare team's beliefs and values regarding care and treatment, etc. The specific meaning of the term 'innovation' was explored earlier in this chapter under clinical practice development.

## Analysis of environmental and user factors

The second essential factor for effective implementation of change is whether the particular practice setting is suitable and ready for the change. It might not be 'ripe for change' if there is extensive resistance to change by the employees or in the team where change is to be implemented. An inappropriate time would be when there are too many unresolved issues or too many unfilled vacancies. There could also be barriers to change, which implies that organisational factors such as funding levels, politics or management are likely to present as obstacles.

In addition to the environment where change will be implemented, another essential component to consider for effective change implementation is the 'users' of the change. Rogers and Shoemaker (1971) identified six categories of users who are likely to be found in the organisation when change is envisaged. They are:

- *Innovators* – individuals who feel excited by novel practices that appear more effective and efficient.
- *Early adopters* – those who accept the change quite soon.
- *Early majority* – the first group to follow the early adopters.
- *Later majority* – other groups join the adopters of the change.
- *Laggards* – individuals who tend to lag behind.
- *Rejecters* – individuals who usually reject any change.

## Innovators, laggards and rejecters

**What, if anything, can practice managers do about each group of staff identified in the above categorisation of users of change?**

Think Point 5.3

Healthcare managers can react or proact in specific ways towards each group of staff for managing the particular change effectively. For instance, with:

- *Innovators* – use the energy, allocate responsibilities; maybe appoint as change agent (leader of the change).
- *Early adopters* – recognise their motivation.
- *Early majority* – give sustained time and support.
- *Later majority* – reinforce by recognition and showing keen interest.
- *Laggards* – give extra support, prevent disillusionment.
- *Rejectors* – line manager to explore, as the individual might have evidence to the contrary, or might, for instance, be experiencing transient personal problems.

### Preparation for the change
A change agent is usually appointed to advocate and lead the implementation of the change. He or she has certain fundamental functions such as:

- To have thorough knowledge of the change envisaged.
- To identify the exact goals of the change.
- To articulate the vision.
- To develop strategies for introducing the change.

- To disseminate relevant knowledge and strategies to appropriate individuals and groups.
- To establish and maintain a working relationship with change users.
- To retain big picture focus while dealing with specifics (integrative thinking).

Sullivan and Decker (2009) indicate that change agents have to be proactive at every step of the change process, and must be able to invest time, effort and energy. They suggest that some of the characteristics that successful change agents should cultivate and master are:

- Well-developed interpersonal and human relations skills.
- Being a role model for the users of the change.
- Being trustworthy.
- Being flexible and persevering.
- Realistic thinking.
- The ability to combine ideas from unconnected sources.
- The ability to energise others.
- The ability to handle resistance.

Thus, change agents have to demonstrate leadership abilities, and the transformational leadership style is particularly relevant for managing change. Some of the key facets of this style compared to those of the frequently demonstrated transactional style are presented in Table 5.2.

Transactional leadership involves the orderly breaking down of tasks but this often leads to loss of vision and energy. On the other hand, transformational leaders keep a distance, take a strategic or 'helicopter' view of the whole picture, lead by being passionate about the task in hand and empower.

## Strategies for implementing the change

Strategies for change can be derived from existing models of change incorporating planned and systematic actions, based on underpinning beliefs and philosophies. As the change agent, there is a range of strategies that the

**TABLE 5.2**    Transactional and transformational leadership

| Transactional | Transformational |
|---|---|
| Is task centred | Empowers relevant others |
| Has a short-/medium-term focus | Inspires by vision |
| Coaches and exercises sheltered learning | Has a long-term focus |
| Rewards formally | Challenges |
| Is comfortable, orderly | Sees home and work lives on a continuum |
| Separates home and work | Rewards informally, personally |
| | Is emotional and passionate |
| | Simplifies and clarifies |

**TABLE 5.3**   Forcefield analysis – named nurse

| Driving forces | Restraining forces |
|---|---|
| Compatible with the government's patients' charter | Could feel threatened |
| | Shifts – practicality |
| Patient choice ascertained | Time factor |
| Follow-up care – admission to discharge | Staff disappointment, frustration |
| Sense of responsibility and autonomy for nurses | Patient may not like the nurse |
| | Patients/relatives frustrated/antagonised if nurse off-duty |
| Direction for nurses | Dissemination of information, e.g. at ward rounds |

mentor can choose from to implement change. One of the first steps in this venture is to do a SWOT or a 'forcefield' analysis. SWOT analyses were introduced in Chapter 4, and an example of a forcefield analysis is presented in Table 5.3.

---

## Activity 5.5   How is change managed?

Consider, maybe in a small group of healthcare professionals working in different specialisms, any one of the changes identified in response to Activity 5.1, for example self-rostering or integrated care pathways, one that approximates a real change issue in the practice area of one of the group members. With the chosen change, do a SWOT or forcefield analysis in relation to your own practice area.

---

At times when a change that is to be implemented is contemplated by managers, an electronic (i.e. by email) or paper copy of the change is sent to all whom the change will affect. Generally, comments are invited from the prospective users of the change, and an open meeting might be held to enable users to ask for clarification. However, there are other well-documented systematic change strategies that are available to the healthcare professionals to choose from, the most noteworthy of which are:

1   Lewin's three-stage process;
2   empirical-rational strategy;
3   normative-re-educative strategy;
4   power-coercive strategy;
5   action research;
6   PDSA;
7   combined strategy.

**TABLE 5.4**   Forcefield analysis – introducing flexible hours

| Probable actions | Driving forces | Restraining forces | Probable actions |
|---|---|---|---|
| ← | What people want | Long-term staff against | → |
| ← | Retention issues | Fear of coming off worse | → |
| ← | Encourage recruitment | 'Unfair' | → |
| ← | Staff morale | Fitting in with practical routine | → |
| ← | Maximum use of staff time | Not feeling part of the team | → |
| | | Staff morale | → |
| | | Lack of communication | → |

Each of these strategies is based on different assumptions held by the change agent about the people who have to accept and use the change. The appropriate strategies vary according to different situations, and a combination of strategies can be used.

### (a) Lewin's three-stage change strategy

Lewin's (1951) three-stage process of change involves unfreezing the situation, implementing the change, and then refreezing it. This is obviously an extremely simplistic explanation of activities that warrant careful planning and conduct. Unfreezing can be achieved by the SWOT or forcefield analyses just discussed. The implementation of the change is referred to as 'movement', and 'refreezing' refers to sustaining the change.

Following a SWOT or forcefield analysis, the actions that can be taken entail reducing the weaknesses and strengthening the driving forces. A format like the ones presented in Table 5.4 for introducing flexible hours, and in Box 5.3 for peri-operative visiting can be utilised for this.

---

### Box 5.3   SWOT analysis – peri-operative visiting

| SWOT analysis | Probable actions |
|---|---|
| Strengths | |
| • Reduce anxiety | |
| • Patient compliance up | |

*(Continued)*

| (Continued) | |
| --- | --- |
| **SWOT analysis** | **Probable actions** |
| • Less post-operative compliance required<br>• Patient articulates preferences to nursing staff<br>• More interdisciplinary collaboration<br>• Patient divulges more information<br>• Continuity of care<br><br>Weaknesses<br><br>• Resources<br>• Time<br>• Possible lack of knowledge<br>• Too many people disseminating information<br><br>Opportunities<br><br>• Role expansion<br>• Specialist role<br>• Education<br>• Increase cost-effectiveness through patient compliance<br>• Enhance patient care<br><br>Threats<br><br>• Lack of continuity of care<br>• Cost – funding<br>• Patient information overload<br>• Elitism – conflict | |

## (b) Empirical-rational strategy

The empirical-rational strategy is used by the change agent by enabling the prospective users of the change to appreciate research findings or other evidence that indicates the need for change. It builds on the assumption that people are essentially rational, are guided by reason, and that if they can be helped to understand the reasons and processes of the proposed change, they are more likely to adopt it. Therefore this strategy is also based on empowerment through giving knowledge. Government health warnings are often based on this strategy.

## (c) Normative-re-educative strategy

Some change topics necessitate predominantly a re-educative approach in that if the users of the change are unfamiliar with the novel idea, then acquisition of new knowledge and skills will be a prerequisite for the change. This approach is also based on the belief that individuals and groups are inherently seeking and accepting novel ways of practising their trade based on evidence or research.

Change has to come from within the organisation, and if the bulk of the organisation's employees see change as a normal process (i.e. the normative strategy prevails) then this also comprises the bottom–up approach that includes the employees' active involvement in planning, implementation and evaluation of the process of change. Such involvement, in turn, leads to increases in motivation and personal growth, alongside commitment and co–operation.

## (d) Power-coercive strategy

Another strategy for implementing change is the power-coercive strategy, in which the change agent emphasises their position power by underlining political and economic dynamics to achieve the desired outcomes and, where necessary, the use of moral power, playing on feelings of guilt and shame. Coercion refers to very strong persuasion to accept the change and may incorporate potential threats and sanctions.

The assumption is that those in control of the organisation will identify the need for change, and people with less power will comply with their plans. If an empirical-rational approach does not work then a power-coercive strategy might be used but this does not usually prove as productive in the long term.

## (e) Action research

As noted earlier, one of the steps that could be considered in the management of change is trialability, i.e. whether a pilot project could be undertaken before full implementation. Change also presents an opportunity for research, i.e. a more systematic implementation of the change along with a more rigorous evaluation of the impact of the change. Thus, practice development can be implemented and evaluated more systematically through action research rather than limiting the implementation at evaluation and sustaining stages of the RAPSIES framework.

## (f) Plan–Do–Study–Act (PDSA)

PDSA is a relatively recent notion that is advocated in the context of service improvement (Institute of Healthcare Improvement (IHI), 2010) in healthcare which is utilised as a strategy for implementation of change that acts as a spiral of continuous evaluation and improvement. Plan, do, study (or check) and act are cardinal steps in this strategy for managing change, and although this may initially sound a simplistic framework, each step entails a number of structured action points. See also Chapter 8 for PDSA as a framework for evaluation.

## Strategy for change

It is likely that during your early years as a newly qualified healthcare profes-sional you were involved in some component of change. This encounter may have been deliberate or incidental. The change may have been initiated through internal or external forces. In relation to this, consider how:

- you reacted to the change;
- you as an individual (or within a group) accepted or resisted the change.;
- you perceived any specific strategy used to bring about the change (e.g. power-coercive, action research, etc.).

### (g) Combined strategy

An appropriate combination of the above six strategies may be structured to suit the innovation, the environment, the users and the change agent.

The concepts of practice development, and change and innovations are widely discussed at national levels mainly at conferences, and through bench-marking. Binnie and Titchen (1999) refer to these activities as a series of journeys, implying that awareness of new ways of working and change man-agement are naturally evolving dimensions within healthcare professions. They also identify a number of principles for practice development, which include components such as promoting and supporting a climate in which work is experienced as intellectually stimulating, growth is fostered and the relevant infrastructure is well developed.

### Implementation of the change

Various factors need to be considered with regards to the actual implementation of the change, e.g. the start date, the evaluation dates, the key staff, any specific paperwork required, if an action research strategy is being employed, how to deal with arising issues, infrastructure and whether all required resources are available, whether users have had the required training, and even if a buddying system is instituted. Dissemination of the impact of the programme is also an option.

### Evaluation of the impact of the change

Naturally, an aspect of healthcare cannot be introduced without instant and continuing evaluation of its effects, and therefore the formative and summative evaluation points should be identified. Models and frameworks for evaluation are discussed in Chapter 8 of this book.

### Sustaining the change

One of the key reasons why many new ideas fail sometime after implemen-tation is shortcomings in the resources needed to sustain the change. Staff motivation also needs to be sustained by reinforcement from the change agent or line managers. Personnel involved in ensuring success of the change should be explicitly recognised, and rewarded as appropriate. The structure, process and outcome mechanism (Donabedian, 1988) should be kept firmly in mind to identify any weak spots in each of these components that need immediate action.

## Mentors as Role Models of EBP and Practice Development

In summarising the discussion on the mentor's role as evidence-based practitioner and practice developer, it very much looks like one of the added values or knock-on effects of the mentor's activities as a practice developer is that it is a suitable dimension for the mentor to embody the qualities of a model healthcare professional. Being amenable to adopting changing modes of clinical interventions that benefit or enhance the health of patients or service users is a characteristic of a role model that mentees can emulate.

Price and Price (2009) support the argument that role modelling is an appropriate method or process for enabling students to learn safe and effective practice. The notion is based on Bandura's (1997) social learning theory which, as noted in Chapter 1, suggests that individuals learn behaviour through observation, mental retention of the procedure utilised, reproducing the behaviour and reinforcement. An analysis of role modelling was also presented in Chapter 1.

Wright and Carrese (2002) conducted a study to ascertain the characteristics of role models in a healthcare profession, and concluded that 'clinical attributes' is one of the most important characteristics, other characteristics being personal qualities (e.g. positive outlook and interpersonal skills) and teaching skills. Paice et al. (2002) explored the significance of doctors as role models for medical students, and report that 'excellent' role models show:

- Positive attitude towards junior colleagues
- Compassion for patients
- Integrity
- Clinical competence
- Enthusiasm for their clinical specialism
- Communication and teaching ability
- Understanding of the importance of the doctor–patient relationship
- Consideration of psychosocial aspects, i.e. viewing the patient as a whole

## Chapter Summary

This chapter has focused on the mentor's role in evidence-based effective practice and clinical practice development, as well as management of change, and has therefore examined:

- Effective practice and clinical effectiveness, and their relevance for the mentor role.
- Evidence-based practice, addressing what it is and how it is achieved; research-based practice, and the mentor's role in identifying, evaluating, applying and disseminating research findings, and how to overcome barriers to implementation.
- Clinical practice development, what the term means, including a concept analysis of practice development, the reasons for developing practice and how they can be managed effectively.
- Managing change, incorporating the key reasons for constant changes in healthcare, and the components necessary for effective change implementation utilising a seven-step framework for doing so systematically, which includes different strategies for implementing change.

## Further Optional Reading

Various detailed examples of innovations and practice development in healthcare are available on the NHS III and the Department of Health website, e.g.:

- Department of Health (2010d) *Quality, Innovation, Productivity and Prevention (QIPP) – Case Studies*. Available at: www.dh.gov.uk/en/Healthcare/Qualityandproductivity/DH_ 118202. Accessed 31 August 2010.

See the following book that asks: 'Is evidence-based practice really best practice?' The book presents a supplementary perspective to the scientific but often mechanical approach that evidence-based practice takes, and re-emphasises the humanistic values that must underpin the art of health and social care practice:

- McCarthy, J. and Rose, P. (2010) *Values-Based Health and Social Care – Beyond Evidence-Based Practice*. London: Sage Publications.

For a website that draws on almost all acceptable databases for all groups of health and social care professionals, see:

- NHS Evidence (2010) *Sources of Information*. Available at: www.evidence.nhs.uk/ aboutus/Pages/SelectingInformationSources.aspx. Accessed 29 July 2010.

A good resource for how to critically appraise research papers is:

- Greenhalgh, T. (2006) *How to Read a Paper: The Basics of Evidence-Based Medicine*. Oxford: BMJ Books.

# 6

# Assessing the Learner's Knowledge and Competence

## Introduction

One of the most fundamental functions of the mentor is to assess students' and other learners' clinical skills and associated knowledge. Assessment is an integral part of all credit awarding healthcare courses, and one of the principal purposes of mentoring courses is to equip course participants with the capability to assess learners' competencies. At the end of each assessment the mentor makes a decision regarding whether the learner is competent to perform each skill independently, unsupervised and safely, and signs the appropriate section of the learner's competency booklet as pass or fail.

There are a number of factors that the mentor needs to take into consideration to fulfil their assessment function effectively. These factors are explored in this chapter from the perspectives of what are assessments, why do we perform them and when, who performs them, and the range of methods of assessment that are available. The specified procedures that have to be followed, and the validity and reliability of assessments are other components that are addressed. These points essentially comprise the principles and processes of assessments. Problems with assessments, as well as past and present criticisms and how they can be averted or resolved, are components addressed in Chapter 7.

In its specification of competence and outcomes for the mentor under 'Assessment and accountability', the NMC (2008a: 52–3) indicates that the mentor should be competent to 'assess learning in order to make judgements related to the NMC standards of proficiency for entry to the register or for recording a qualification at a level above initial registration'. The outcomes of this particular mentor competence are:

- To foster professional growth, personal development and accountability through support of students in practice.
- To demonstrate a breadth of understanding of assessment strategies and ability to contribute to the total assessment process as part of the teaching team.
- To provide constructive feedback to students and assist them in identifying future learning needs and actions, manage failing students so that they may enhance their performance and capability for safe and effective practice or be able to understand their failure and the implications of this for their future.
- To be accountable for confirming that students have met the NMC or not met the NMC competencies in practice and as a sign-off mentor confirm that students have met or not met the NMC standards of proficiency and are capable of safe and effective practice.

The concepts that are inherent to the principles of assessment implicated in the above NMC outcomes are therefore essential, and are addressed in this chapter.

## Chapter outcomes

On completion of this chapter, you should be able to:

1   Identify what assessments are, and the elements of healthcare courses on which students are assessed.
2   Enunciate a number of reasons for assessment of clinical skills and knowledge of students on healthcare profession courses.
3   Cite instances of various staff members who are involved in assessment, including the roles of self- and peer assessment.
4   Explain a range of strategies that mentors can utilise in the conduct of student assessments, and the various key principles of assessments that they need to abide by to fulfil this function.
5   Explain the role of 'ongoing record of achievement' and the requirements that the mentor has to fulfil to be able to sign off proficiency competently.
6   Explain the processes of the management of assessment of clinical competencies, and how assessments can meet essential criteria such as validity and reliability.

## What are Assessments?

To begin to examine the principles and processes of assessments, it is useful to establish first what you as the healthcare professional already know about assessments of competencies.

> ## Activity 6.1   What you already know about assessments
>
> 1 Think of the courses that you have already attended, and any one(s) you might currently be on. Think also of your contact with learners and students on various programmes of study. What are the various methods of assessment that are used to assess learners' knowledge and skills? Jot down as many methods as you can think of.
> 2 Consider what else you already know about assessments, which aspects of assessments you are unclear about, and what else you feel you need to know about assessments. Make written notes of your responses.

So what do you already know about assessments? In response to Activity 6.1, you may have thought that assessment of clinical skills is best carried out by direct observation of the learner's performance, and some by reflective practice write-ups. Essays and written examinations are used for the assessment of theory. Most of these will be examined in this chapter under 'how to assess'.

Examples of assessments of theory and practice in healthcare education programmes include:

- structured essays;
- objective or multiple-choice tests;
- profiles and portfolio, and reflective write-ups;
- practice-based competencies;
- care or case studies;
- seminars;
- written examination;
- OSCE (i.e. Objective Structured/Simulated Clinical Examination);
- short-answer questions;
- practical assessments in skills laboratories;
- individually negotiated projects;
- longitudinal studies.

Your response to what else you feel you need to know about assessments obviously depends very much on your experience, existing knowledge and understanding of the concept, and it varies between individuals. You might have felt, for instance, that you could do with knowing more about formative, summative, continuous, peer/self-assessment, or about practice competencies.

## What do we mean by assessments?

A number of assessment methods such as written examinations, practical assessments and projects have just been identified.

---

### Activity 6.2    Assessments I've passed

To explore this area further, first look back to a course you attended, preferably recently, and make notes on the following:

A list of assessments that you had to pass to complete the course successfully. When exactly during the course were you assessed, and on which components of the course?
Specifically what was assessed?

---

If you were assessed by continuous assessment, then you would have been exposed to a range of assessment components on different occasions, during both practice placements and in university skill laboratories and classrooms.

### *Definitions of assessment*

The dictionary (Brown, 2002: 331) states that the word 'assess' originates from the Latin word *assidere*, which means sit by or beside, which implies a close relationship and sharing an experience. The word also means 'estimate the extent, value or worth' of something. Therefore, assessment tends to imply staying by the learner's side and observing them perform a clinical skill with a view to stating at the end of the performance whether the skill was carried out competently. It also seems to imply being supportive and identifying subsequent learning needs.

Taking a step back, however, it is important to note that an assessment is not an activity we perform only occasionally to fulfil our work role. We assess life situations all the time before we take any action, whether it is to do with assessing whether to wear a coat when going out based on the perceived weather and temperature outside, whether it is safe to overtake when driving, or whether we can treat ourselves to a delicious cake while bearing in mind the day's calorie intake. Such assessments do not result in someone awarding us a pass or fail but they still involve assessing stimuli or data, and then making a decision.

Assessment is also reflected in patient assessment, which entails collecting information and identifying actual and potential patient problems from the data, from which decisions are made regarding the actions to be taken. Student assessment, however, is related to collecting information as evidence of the student's ability to perform particular clinical skills or competencies. Some of the core skills necessary for assessing patients' needs and problems are also relevant for assessing learners. These are observing, measuring, interviewing and making decisions. These skills also apply to assessment of students' knowledge and skills. For assessing health profession learners' clinical competencies and related knowledge, assessment can be defined as the purposeful observation and questioning undertaken to ascertain the learner's ability to perform particular clinical interventions in precise accordance with established or approved guidelines, and their knowledge of rationales for each action. Curzon (2003) suggests that assessments involve collecting, measuring and interpreting information related to students' responses to the process of instruction.

Other definitions are provided by Nicklin and Kenworthy (2000), for instance, who define assessment as a measurement that directly relates to the quality and quantity of learning and is therefore concerned with students' progress and attainment. While quantity of learning could imply the number of skills or part skills that the learner has already learnt, quality of learning refers to how thoroughly the skills have been learnt. The latter would also suggest progress and identifying areas of further learning.

### What do we assess?

The NMC's (2010a) *Standards for Pre-registration Nursing Education* identifies the exact 'generic' competencies and 'field' (previously known as 'branch') competencies that each student needs to achieve to gain registered nurse status on the NMC's professional register. There are also 'specialist practitioner outcomes' for SCPHNs (NMC, 2004c), for instance, as there are criteria, competence and outcomes for mentors and practice teachers (NMC, 2008a). Similarly, the HPC publishes separate standards for pre-qualifying different AHP courses. These standards and competencies are reflected in the course and modules' aims and learning outcomes, in theory and in practice components.

The UKCC (1999) advocated an outcomes-based competency approach to education which encourages the development of knowledge, understanding, practical and technical skills, attitudes and values. Current pre-registration nurse education curricula thus contain generic and field (mental health, adult, child and learning disabilities) competencies under four 'domains': (i) professional values; (ii) communication and interpersonal skills; (iii) nursing practice and decision making; and (iv) leadership, management and teamworking for entry to the professional register (NMC, 2010a), as noted in Chapter 2. The NMC (2010a) standards will be implemented from 2011, and therefore the preceding NMC (2004a) standards of proficiency remain current until at least 2014. These NMC standards document can be accessed through the NMC's website, and it is advisable for nurse mentors to print and keep a copy for reference purposes.

As we will see later, it is absolutely vital for the mentor to establish very early on during the practice placement exactly which specific competencies they are expected to assess students on during that particular placement. Otherwise, the assessment may not meet the curriculum requirements. In the notes you made in response to Activity 6.2, you may have mentioned that the NMC has already laid down the components that we need to assess in the form of competencies, but more detailed information can usually be found in a range of documents such as the student's course assessment booklet, the assessor's handbook and the course curriculum.

In addition to the NMC's (2010a) generic and field competencies, essential skills clusters are incorporated into all pre-registration nursing education programmes, and the specific ones that form part of particular practice placement practice objectives to be achieved by students are discussed with them and their mentors before students embark on the particular placement.

All assessments of the pre-registration curriculum are mandatory, and those in the first year of the programme are set at academic level 4 (or level C – certificate level); those for Year 2 are set at level 5 (level I – Intermediate or diploma level), and those for Year 3 at level 5 or 6 (level H – Honours degree level) depending on whether the student is following a diploma or a degree programme (QAA, 2008). Level 7 (Masters level), and level 8 (Doctoral level) are also identified by the QAA. Various other ways of differentiating between academic levels have also already been developed (e.g. Steinaker and Bell, 1979; Krathwohl, 2002).

The competencies booklet given to students contains other useful information such as the process of assessment, the roles and responsibilities of the mentor, those of the student, and the university support available to them.

## Optional activity – Pre-registration student assessment

Find out from your partner university all the assessments that the pre-registration student needs to pass for the field-specific part of the programme while on placement in your practice setting. You could access this information via the link tutor, for instance, for your practice setting.

In addition to the placement competencies or practice objectives set by the university, students are encouraged to achieve as many other competencies as the placement can offer and thereby maximise learning. A number of clinical areas have their own clearly identified competencies or learning objectives that can be achieved during placement. A number of them are optional for pre-registration students but compulsory for newly appointed qualified healthcare professionals on induction or preceptee programmes.

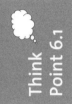

**Think Point 6.1**

## Practice placement competencies

Obtain a copy of the competencies or learning objectives for your practice area, and consider:

Are these learning objectives separate from ward or team aims and objectives? If so, why?
How far do the learning objectives give a clear indication of all competencies that students can learn during the placement?

The competencies are usually available in a 'learning resources' folder for students in your practice setting but it might prove useful to obtain a photocopy of this for yourself for revisiting if required.

In addition to the regulatory bodies' standards of proficiency, professional bodies such as the Chartered Society of Physiotherapy (2002) publish further specific standards, such as those in the *Curriculum Framework for Qualifying Programmes in Physiotherapy*, for instance. This document identifies the nine outcomes that physiotherapy students have to achieve by the time they complete their preparatory programme, along with further guidelines. It specifies that, on successful completion of a recognised programme, graduates should be able to demonstrate their capacity to:

- practise within the core areas of physiotherapy;
- manage themselves and work with others to optimise results;
- enable people to optimise their health and social well-being;
- deliver physiotherapy in response to individual need;
- promote equality to all in physiotherapy practice;
- demonstrate and apply knowledge and understanding to issues affecting physiotherapy practice;
- engage in research and evidence-based healthcare;
- respond appropriately to changing demands;
- practise and promote CPD.

## Why do We Need to Assess our Students?

We have already referred to some of the aims of assessments. Most individuals have mixed feelings about being assessed, as on the one hand, it creates anxiety, but on the other hand, on passing the assessment, the assessee can be given permission to practise the particular clinical skill without close supervision. To begin our discussion on why we need to assess, consider what the range of purposes of assessments is, in addition to the (NMC, 2008a) requirement for mentors to assess learners.

---

## Activity 6.3   Purposes of assessments

Think of all the methods of assessment you noted during Activity 6.1, and of the reasons for assessing students and other learners. Make notes of these reasons for assessment. What did each assessment test?

---

As noted at the beginning of the chapter, according to the NMC, the mentor must indicate that the student has achieved the NMC (2010a) standards for pre-registration nurse education in that they are safe and effective in practice, and thus the practice competencies are designed to test the student's ability to perform clinical patient care skills. Structured essays test the student's knowledge and understanding of concepts in nursing. In addition to these, assessments also ascertain learning in the affective domain (Bloom, 1956; discussed in Chapter 3), that is, values and attitudes. Several purposes of assessments are identified by different writers. In summary, we assess learners:

- To establish and then authorise them as developing health professionals, to practise specific clinical skills without close supervision.
- To inform the learner of their level of achievement at that point in time.
- To determine the student's progress with the learning programme.
- To ascertain the learner's overall competence and fitness for practice.
- To motivate the learner towards new components of learning.
- To judge the level of professional learning in the cognitive (knowledge and thinking), psychomotor (dexterity with clinical skills), and affective (attitude) components.
- For the student to identify further learning needs based on self-assessment and mentor feedback.

As assessments also constitute an opportunity for identifying learning needs, this suggests that learning is an integral component of the assessment process, and not simply a means of measuring attainment. Students are encouraged to undertake self-assessment and to reflect on their learning. It could be argued that all assessments are learning situations, in that if the assessee makes any error, then they are likely to be aware of it, or the assessor will point it out to them and identify learning needs. This notion also suggests that even if the student performs the skill competently, there is still scope for progressing from 'competent' to 'proficient' levels, for instance, and subsequently to 'expert' on Benner's (2001) skill acquisition continuum.

From the teacher's perspective, assessments also provide a measure of teaching effectiveness. It provides some feedback on the mentor's and their colleagues' effectiveness at teaching particular competencies during practice placements. Naturally, the student will normally have had some teaching related to those competencies at the university beforehand. Assessments of theory also provide nurse lecturers with some measure of their university-based teaching.

In addition to the aims of assessments already mentioned, another function of assessments is to fulfil one of society's needs directly, in that they identify which healthcare professionals have acquired the necessary repertoire of knowledge and competencies for safe and competent practice, as a primary practitioner initially, and probably as a specialist later.

## Who Assesses Learners?

As to who assesses learners, obviously it is qualified healthcare professionals who have completed a mentoring course who are given 'a licence' to assess learners' competencies. However, it is pertinent to consider the broader question of who else are the relevant personnel who assess competencies.

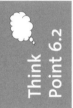

**Think Point 6.2**

## Who assesses?

Think about assessments you and your colleagues have been involved in recently. Spend a few minutes thinking about who conducted the assessments, on what, on whom and how. Is it only the mentor who assesses the learner's competencies, or are other individuals also afforded this responsibility?

Perhaps an immediate response to this Think Point is that it is the mentor who assesses, or teams of mentors. However, the NMC (2008a) indicates that assessments are also performed by other registrants, practice teachers and qualified teachers. In fact, you might have concluded that all qualified healthcare professionals, including doctors, are involved in assessments, albeit often informally or indirectly. So, the answer to the question 'Who assesses?' could be everyone in the practice setting, but includes students' self-assessment, peer assessment, and assessment by patients or service users. These are now discussed.

## Student self-assessment

Self-assessment is one of the most valuable forms of assessment for students. It is almost always formative and therefore a learning exercise. As implied, the student uses a set of criteria or a checklist, written or mental, to self-assess their knowledge of a sub-topic area or of a specific competency. It also enables them to own the learning and to control the way they meet their needs. Self-assessment may be performed informally or more formally by the use of profiling documents or reflective diaries.

Much informal or subconscious self-assessment carried out by learners is based on their own individual aspirations, values and beliefs. These could be influenced by their views on patient or service-user care based on their own personal and professional experiences.

---

### Activity 6.4    Self-assessment

Take a critical look at the idea of self-assessment by students, and of the strengths and weaknesses of self-assessments, and identify as many of these as you can think of.

---

What is self-assessment? Falchikov (1986) states that in self-assessment the learner judges their own performance against their own assessment criteria. According to Boud (1991), self-assessment is characterised by involvement of students in identifying standards and/or criteria to apply to their work and making judgements about the extent to which they have met them.

On examining the concept with groups of post-registration students, a number of areas of strengths as well as weaknesses were identified (Gopee, 2000) – see Table 6.1.

**TABLE 6.1**   The strengths and weaknesses of self-assessment

| Strengths | Weaknesses |
|---|---|
| Inspires a conscious effort to be honest with self | Student can be too strict or too lenient |
| Opportunity to identify limitations of own knowledge, and of learning needs | Self-assessment is subjective, and student may be unaware of the perceptions of relevant others |
| Identify where more practice/knowledge gain is required | Students may be unable to gauge the effectiveness of own performance |
| Is less traumatic than traditional methods of assessment such as examinations | Students can be too self-critical |
|  | May worsen a student's poor self-image |

*Source*: Gopee, 2000

## Peer assessment

The value and impact of peers' and colleagues' impressions of our competence in various aspects of our roles cannot be underestimated. This is often
informal, with colleagues, friends and even family members having different
perceptions of our capability, based perhaps on their different professional
experiences.

Because of its value to the student, increasingly peer assessment is being built
into formal assessment processes. In distance and e-learning modes of education delivery, facilitators often encourage students to form their own 'learning
sets' for the purposes of learning together, discussions and questioning each
other. Peer assessment, in this case, is not formal in that other students or colleagues do not usually award a summative 'pass' or 'fail' to the peer assessed.
They do, however, provide valuable opinions and feedback on the individual's
knowledge, which can be formally incorporated into a profile or a record of
reflective learning. In this way, peer assessment usually presents an opportunity
to verbalise uncertainties and reservations about one's learning without having
to deal with the anxiety of examinations and pass or fail situations.

Assessment by peers, formal or informal, is increasingly becoming accepted
as an educationally sound activity. Many of us may find assessing our peers
uncomfortable. We either do not wish to appear to be over-critical, and
therefore tend not to assess or voice our views fully, or we feel that as we have
such good rapport with our peers, we could damage their self-confidence
with our 'criticisms'. It is also important to recognise that being assessed by
our peer group can be more daunting than being assessed by a qualified assessor. If it is done badly, peer assessment can quickly destroy students' confidence or make them feel unable to face their peers again.

Peer assessment, therefore, just like any other form of assessment, can benefit from the expertise of a facilitator if it is to be effective and help the student. Thus, peers who are doing the assessing, as well as the person being
assessed, are helped by the facilitator to recognise the parameters of their roles.
However, as with self-assessment, there can well be problematic areas related
to peer assessment – Table 6.2 identifies quite a few of the advantages and
disadvantages.

Another related term is *peer review*, which involves seeking the views and
impressions of peers in a structured or semi-structured way. When clinicians
design a new protocol or audit tool, for instance, they may ask an uninvolved
colleague who works some distance away but in the same clinical specialism
to comment on it prior to finalisation for use. Lecturers usually have to ask
a colleague to observe their teaching on specified occasions and provide
feedback against particular criteria.

**TABLE 6.2**  Advantages and disadvantages of peer assessment

| Advantages of peer assessment | Disadvantages of peer assessment |
| --- | --- |
| Confirms previously held belief in skills or lack of them | Some can find it hard to take any criticism from equals |
| Provides clarity to self-assessment findings | Increased anxiety |
| Chance to share colleagues' experiences | Someone can be over-critical, and destructive |
| Identifying problems | Can be judgemental about the person |
| Receiving feedback | Takes so much effort and resulting anxiety that pointed out weaknesses may not be fully taken on board |
| Feedback from colleagues/students of equal status has impact | May not be supportive enough |
| Opportunity to practise the skill | The individual might not accept peers' views |
| Is formative, i.e. is not a pass/fail mark for the course | Facilitators' knowledge of relevant literature, research, etc. may be limited |
|  | Can destroy self-confidence, and lead to deserting the venture/vocation altogether |
|  | Disagreement between peers |
|  | Availability of opportunities/peers for peer assessment |
|  | Lack of commitment |

*Source*: Gopee, 2001

## Patient or service user involvement in assessment of competencies

One of the judges of how competently a healthcare profession learner performs a clinical skill could be the patient or service user. User involvement in learner assessment and providing feedback on how competently the learner functioned in particular care interventions is increasingly advocated by regulatory bodies (e.g. NMC, 2006b). In recommending user involvement in assessments, the NMC (2006b, 2010a) advises HEIs to explore ways in which lay people (including service users and carers) can be involved in the assessment of practice, and supply evidence of this involvement, and of that of clinical practitioners in Programme Boards/Boards of Study that establish the requirements for practice learning and assessment (Mott MacDonald, 2009).

So, what are the specific ways in which the mentor can do this? Usually, the mentor gauges how content the patient or service user is with the care they receive by observation, and even by casually asking them. The patient or service user can provide feedback to the mentor about the assessee's communication skills, injection-giving skills, and teaching relaxation skills, for example, which are competencies under the NMC (2010a) domains communication and interpersonal skills, nursing practice and decision-making, and leadership, management and teamworking, respectively. User involvement in

assessment of competencies under the domain professional values can be
achieved by the mentor asking the patient or service user if they felt that their
consent had been obtained by the student prior to the clinical intervention,
if they felt that they were treated with dignity and whether confidentiality
was maintained in the presence of others.

Evidence of effective service user involvement in students' learning and
assessment prevail (e.g. Gutteridge and Dobbins, 2010; Stickley et al., 2010),
although it is acknowledged that it is a time–intensive activity that also
requires additional infrastructure.

## How are Assessments Conducted?

Learners deemed competent in performing a particular clinical skill can move
on to learn other skills identified as their practice objectives for the placement. In this major section on how to assess, further principles of assessment
are addressed, and comprise:

- ensuring the mentee has learned the clinical skill;
- the assessor's essential interpersonal skills;
- dimensions of assessment;
- levels of assessment;
- fairness of assessment;
- pass or fail decisions and performance criteria.

Additionally, the process of assessment of competencies has to be managed,
decisions made and feedback given to the assessee. These latter points, along
with how the mentor averts and resolves problems of assessment, are examined in Chapter 7.

### Ensuring the mentee has learned the clinical skill

An important prerequisite of assessment of a learner is to ensure that they
have been taught the clinical skill systematically and given the necessary practice opportunities over time and under supervision prior to the point of
assessment. What skills, competence and competencies are was discussed in
Chapter 2, and how learners acquire the required competencies, including
stages and levels of skill acquisition (e.g. Fitts and Posner, 1973; Steinaker and
Bell, 1979; Benner, 2001), in Chapter 3. But crucially and logically, before the
student is asked to demonstrate that they are competent in any skill, they
naturally need to learn to perform the skill according to approved procedures,
and under the guidance of a registrant. The learning also has to be in the

context of eventualities in the practice setting (i.e. situated learning – e.g. Phillips et al., 2000).

## The assessor's essential interpersonal skills

Assessment is a role that has to be executed responsibly by the mentor, and to do so effectively, certain specific personal and interpersonal skills are essential to enable the student to feel at ease when they are being assessed performing clinical interventions.

---

### Activity 6.5    Interpersonal skills in assessing a student

Make a list of what you consider to be the general communication skills required in all assessment situations, and then a list of the more specific communication skills required by the mentor for conducting assessments effectively.

---

Several communication skill items emerge when exploring in detail what and how the mentor communicates with the assessee. Box 6.1 lists many of the essential interpersonal skills that are required during assessments, identified by just one group of registrants on a mentor course.

---

### Box 6.1    Communication and interpersonal factors related to assessments

**Generic communication skills**

- Non-verbal communication – e.g. eye contact, facial expression
- Body language – posture, body orientation, proximity, attitude, behaviour, space
- Being non-judgemental – warmth, empathy, respect

**Specific interpersonal skills**

- Putting the assessee at ease
- Enabling assessee to relax if anxious so that they can perform the skill to their potential
- Building confidence by positive feedback if necessary
- Giving clear directions
- Continuous feedback

*(Continued)*

*(Continued)*

| Generic communication skills | Specific interpersonal skills |
|---|---|
| • Always remaining calm | • Being non-judgemental by not criticising verbally or non-verbally |
| • Openness | |
| • Questioning – open or closed questions | • Giving prompts/clues if student's mind goes blank |
| • Reflecting | • Allowing enough time for the learner to perform the skill fully |
| • Active listening | |
| • Verbal communication – pace, volume, tone, clarity | • Making time to listen, and to maintain rapport |
| • Diplomacy | • Preventing observer bias and observer effect |
| • Considering environmental factors | • Ascertaining level of understanding of terminologies/ jargon |
| • Being enthusiastic, interested | |
| • Making time, using silence | |
| • Constructive criticism/advice | • Confidence – in the student/in self |
| • Approachable and friendly, non-intimidatory | • Reinforcing what has been discussed |

## Dimensions of assessment

There are a number of other essential facets of assessments that we need to consider to gain a more comprehensive picture of how to assess. Quinn and Hughes (2007) and others identify what is generally known as dimensions of assessments. Particularly relevant are whether assessments are:

1   continuous or episodic;
2   formative or summative;
3   criterion-referenced or norm-referenced.

### Continuous or episodic assessments

Until the latter half of the 1980s, the assessment of pre-registration students used to take place at pre-determined points during their course. The student on the general nursing course was assessed on their ability to administer medications in Year 1 of the course, and to use aseptic techniques, and organise the total care of an individual or a group of patients or service users on specific subsequent occasions. They also had to pass written examinations at the end of the course. These are episodic assessments. Obviously, students had to learn numerous other nursing skills necessary to function as a healthcare professional, which were identified in a booklet and signed as appropriate. However, these snapshot assessments were not seen as representing the wide range of skills acquired during placements, nor were they seen as a genuine representation of how students usually delivered care, and they therefore fell into disfavour. They were replaced by continuous assessment and subsequently by modularisation of preparatory programmes, involving assessment of practice and theory on numerous occasions throughout the course.

Episodic (or intermittent) assessments therefore involve testing the student at specific times or occasions during an educational programme, such as at the end of a module, a placement or year. Continuous assessment aims to increase the quality and quantity of evidence gathered in relation to achievement of competencies by each individual student. It involves a continuing awareness by the mentor of the student's level of knowledge and competence, and is thus a cumulative judgement about progress and achievement.

---

## Activity 6.6   Advantages and disadvantages of continuous and episodic assessments

Consider what you think might be the advantages and disadvantages of episodic and continuous assessments, and make some notes.

---

The principal reason for episodic assessments being discredited in nursing and midwifery in the past is that decisions about the student's competence were being made on the basis of one-off performances. This performance, be it excellent or otherwise, might be atypical. Another disadvantage is that some key skills can remain untested if they do not present themselves during the identified assessment episode. Recently, following extensive consultation, the NMC (2010a) has introduced 'progression points' in the pre-registration nursing and midwifery education curriculum when students are assessed and must achieve a 'Pass' on several key competencies before progressing to the subsequent stage of their education programme. These assessments can also be examples of episodic assessment, and students are required to demonstrate that they are competent in those competencies to be able to register subsequently with the NMC as a RN or RM.

### Formative or summative assessments

Another dimension of assessment is whether the assessment is formative or summative. In common with the context of evaluation (which we discuss in

Chapter 8), 'formative' relates to the developmental and improvement stages of something (e.g. a clinical skill). The primary aim of the formative assessment of a professional practice skill is to promote learning so that the learner can perform the skill safely and effectively, and knows the rationales for each step of the intervention. The student's capability is thus developed under conditions in which they can reflect-in-action and think creatively, without being too concerned about final pass or fail grades, and also has the opportunity to take time to learn the skill thoroughly with the support of mentors.

Formative assessment applies to assessment of theory as well as to practical skills. For the theory component of education programmes, the student thereby obtains feedback on the evidence they are presenting to the marker or lecturer on how far they are demonstrating knowledge of the subject area, critical analysis, general presentation of the paper, etc. Formative assessments are therefore instituted to provide feedback to the student on their progress, and their aims are to:

- maximise learning;
- identify strengths/weaknesses;
- inform the student of how they are progressing;
- allow for individual development.

As a concept and an activity, formative assessments have been advocated for decades, but their implementation proves erratic even today, which could be due to them being yet another extra requirement to create time for in busy day-to-day professional activities in both practice setting and HEIs. Thus it has resource and efficiency implications. It is, however, an educationally sound concept and students tends to be grateful for the feedback they receive from them. On exploring the prevalence of its usage in nurse education, Duers and Brown's (2009) study revealed that formative assessments have the 'potential to improve learning so that high quality, safe and effective nursing care to patients may be provided' (2009: 658). Koh (2010) also reports various benefits of formative assessments in nurse education.

'Summative' relates to a point in time during a unit of learning, for example a practice placement, when the mentor makes a decision about whether to declare the learner competent or otherwise on a specific component of learning. They are conducted to determine whether the learner is now competent to work without direct supervision and, if so, then this is recorded in their competencies' booklet.

Summative assessments also constitute a periodic record of the student's achievement of the aims and outcomes of a course or module. The grade awarded for these assessments, along with those for coursework and examinations contribute to the final classification of the student's university award.

It might prove useful to ask your mentee, or to look back on any long course you have done in recent years, and identify the range of formative and summative assignments incorporated in the programme. As to assessment in the practice setting, the student learning part-skills (e.g. some of the skills required for administering an intramuscular injection) itself constitutes a formative assessment. The NMC's (2010b) 'signing off' of competencies point in the pre-registration programme constitutes a summative assessment.

In healthcare courses, summative assessments are concerned with patient or service user safety and standards of practice. They are also concerned with justice for the student and credibility of the university's awards. They must therefore meet the highest standards of reliability and validity, which are discussed in some detail later in this chapter.

### Criterion-referenced or norm-referenced assessments

The third dimension of assessment we consider is norm referencing and criterion referencing. In norm-referenced assessment, the student's score, marks or grades are determined to an extent by those of other students in a given group or cohort. Programme Assessment Boards (also known as Award Boards) have the discretion to adjust the marks required by a particular cohort to achieve a particular grade if unusual circumstances have prevailed. Criterion-referenced assessments are different in that the score or mark given to a particular student for a particular piece of coursework is decided entirely on the basis of a pre-determined set of marking criteria. Students will have been informed of these criteria long before the assessment date.

## Norm- or criterion-referenced assessments

Think about some of the assessments you've mentioned for Activity 6.1 and decide whether they are norm-referenced assessments or criterion-referenced.

Think Point 6.3

Occasionally, a criterion-referenced assessment can be marked on a norm-referenced basis at the discretion of the appropriate Programme Assessment Board.

## Assessing different levels of competence

Student nurses tend to be taught and assessed at different academic levels during Year 1, Year 2 and Year 3. The NMC's (2004a) standards of proficiency and subsequent generic and field competencies noted in Chapter 3 are configured at different academic levels in the competencies booklets that students take to practice placements. Healthcare assistants studying for national vocational qualification are also assessed differently at different levels.

To teach and assess competencies at different levels of learning, a number of current nurse education curricula tend to use Steinaker and Bell's (1979) model (or taxonomy) of experiential learning. This taxonomy consists of exposure level, participation, identification, internalisation and dissemination. A broad guide to how the experiential taxonomy levels can equate with the QAA's (2008) academic levels is:

- Certificate level/academic level 4 – exposure, participation;
- Diploma level/academic level 5 – participation, identification and internalisation;
- Degree level/academic level 6 – identification, internalisation and dissemination.

This is a very simple classification and just a general guide which underpins specific wording of competencies to reflect the different levels. Alternatively, some programmes use Benner's (2001) stages of skill acquisition model, which was discussed in Chapter 2. Others use Bondy's (1983) five levels of competency, namely dependent, marginal, assisted, supervised and independent.

The assessment of theory of nursing at different levels, on the other hand, is usually based on Bloom's (1956) taxonomy of cognitive learning, which was also discussed in Chapter 3. You may wish to look back to the appropriate section to remind yourself of the details of this model, which comprises knowledge, comprehension, application, analysis, synthesis and evaluation. In both models of assessment, the first points, that is, exposure and knowledge, represent lower-level learning and the last points represent the higher levels.

## Fairness of assessments

In assessments, we are measuring the performance of the individual student on particular competencies. Wouldn't you agree, however, that assessments have to be as objective as possible and must be fair to each student? What does 'fairness of assessment' mean?

---

### Activity 6.7   Barriers to 'fairness'

Think about your own experiences of assessment (either assessing or being assessed) and consider instances that can make assessments 'unfair', and how we can make them 'fair'. Identify all factors that you feel interfere with the fairness of the assessment, using the three headings: (a) student factors; (b) mentor factors; and (c) environmental factors. If you can't remember being assessed, then make some notes of your own ideas of what we should be aware of during an assessment to ensure that it is being conducted fairly.

It is conceivable that, on occasion, the demand being made on a student during assessment or the questions being asked may seem beyond the boundaries of what would generally be expected. Fairness of assessment refers to being aware of external circumstances that could influence the student's performance of the clinical skill. There are several factors that could hamper fairness of assessments. An unfair assessment could also mean that it might not be a valid assessment. Student factors that can make an assessment unfair include:

- expected level of knowledge is too high;
- theory–practice disjunction;
- not enough opportunities to practise the competencies;
- last-minute delays or changes;
- undeclared physical illness or fatigue.

You should be able to think of other student factors, including personal circumstances. Mentor factors include the mentor not working on the same shift as their mentee, bias towards or against the student, not having had educational preparation to become a mentor, overpowering attitude, and lack of knowledge of the student's course. Some of the factors in the clinical environment that might unfairly affect assessments are interruptions, lack of resources in the practice setting (e.g. equipment), suitability of placement and low staffing levels.

## Pass or fail decisions and performance criteria

Following a fairly conducted assessment, the mentor has to decide whether it's a pass or a fail for the particular competency. This decision may well depend entirely on whether the student closely followed the trust's approved procedure to perform the clinical skill, or the written (or unwritten) protocol. The procedure is the main form of 'performance criteria'.

### What am I looking for in the student?

Consider two examples of assessment of competence that you may have been involved in. This could be a pre-registration or post-registration course competency.

(a)  How did the mentor determine what criteria to use to pass or fail the learner?
(b)  What influenced them to choose these particular criteria?

Think Point 6.4

The term *performance criteria* refers to the pre-determined set of components that are used for deciding whether the learner performed the clinical skill competently. They can therefore constitute a checklist of the step-by-step actions taken by the assessee when performing the skill. These step-by-step actions are normally the trust's approved procedure or clinical guidelines for that skill, and are set down in two columns as 'actions' and 'rationales', and usually supported by references to make them evidence based. They are normally kept in the practice setting's 'Policies and Procedures' section for use and for reference purposes. There is likely to be a separate folder for clinical guidelines or protocols which refer to expanded role competencies.

The term performance criteria is also used in NVQ programmes but with a slightly different meaning. Quinn and Hughes (2007) refer to them as *performance indicators*. However, for those nursing activities for which there is no identified step-by-step approved procedure, the performance criteria can be established by asking the skilled practitioner to describe to someone in detail everything that they would do to perform the skill competently. For instance, there might not be a procedure for assessing communication skills, for bed-making, for taking body temperature using tympanic thermometers or, say, for doing patient handovers. A set of performance criteria for patient handovers (or 'reporting on patients' progress') is presented in Box 6.2.

---

### Box 6.2   Performance criteria for assessing competency – patient handover

- Have the right documentation, e.g. care plan/pathway, to refer to
- Have a good understanding of the patient's conditions
- State the procedures that have been performed, e.g. removal of drains, sutures, etc.
- Keep the information concise and focused
- Use an appropriate genre of English
- Pitch the amount of information imparted to the level of knowledge the handover recipients already have, e.g. more detailed information may need to be imparted if new staff or students are present, and vice versa
- Ensure that information that must be given, is given
- Inform of individual patient's overall progress
- Note any relevant communication from the patient's family or from members of the multi-disciplinary team
- State any investigation results received, and any subsequent action prescribed
- State any changes in medication, and patient's reaction to them
- State the plan of care for the rest of the day
- Include patient's awareness of own condition, e.g. in mental health
- Observe confidentiality issues, especially for bedside handovers

For competencies for which there are no written performance criteria in the practice setting in the procedures or clinical guidelines folder, they might be found in, for instance, *The Royal Marsden Hospital Manual of Clinical Nursing Procedures* (Dougherty and Lister, 2008). They might also be available from the National Institute of Health and Clinical Excellence (NICE), especially clinical guidelines, via their website or from manufacturers' instructions. As in the trust's procedure, clinical guidelines are usually tabulated as actions and rationales in two columns, and include a references list. However, from the time a book or clinical guideline is written to the time it is available for use, adjustments may have been made to the procedure, based on more up-to-date evidence or research. Trust-based procedures tend to have an addendum to reflect this, which in fact makes them even more up to date than books.

As to keeping the information precise, Castledine (1998), for instance, indicates that handover reports are time limited as they could be seen as keeping healthcare staff away from direct patient care. On noticing ineffective patient handovers practices, Davies and Priestley (2006) suggest that conversation on irrelevant topics should be excluded from this activity. Furthermore, some commentators like Walsh and Ford (1989) see handovers as a ritual, although in reality they comprise a necessary medium for communicating the effects of care and treatment to staff on the next shift.

Depending on the clinical specialism, further specific information may need to be imparted during handovers, for example resuscitation status, mobility levels in rehabilitation services. Very importantly, often teaching and learning points arise from patient handovers, for both students and clinically based unqualified staff and registrants. Thus, the performance criteria for passing or failing a student on their ability to do patient's handover can be quite involved.

## Ongoing Record of Achievement and Signing-Off Proficiency

In its periodic review of pre-registration education curricula, the NMC (2006b) found that mentors wished to have access to their mentees' progress documentation of preceding practice placements as evidence of skills that they are already deemed competent in, prior to establishing the mentee's learning requirements and needs. In response to this, the NMC (2007a) issued guidelines for universities to implement a systematic way of establishing a mechanism to achieve this.

This mechanism was initially termed a 'passport' but due to different interpretations of this term, it was changed to 'ongoing achievement record' (OAR) (it retained at least one element of passports which is to have the student's photograph included in the document). With the OAR identifying the student's 'progress' so far, and the placement's competencies booklet that the student brings with them, a 'diagnostic assessment' of competencies can be made before establishing specific learning needs and objectives at the initial interview at the beginning of the placement. The OAR is a requirement for all students who commenced on pre-registration nurse education programmes in September 2008, following guidance provided by the NMC (2007a).

Consequently, universities issue students with an OAR document with provision for recording their progress throughout their course, which include in particular a record of all their practice placements. The NMC (2007a: 2) notes that the OAR is necessary for maintaining continuity of assessment, to ensure safe and effective practice, and 'enable judgement to be made on the student's progress'. The sign-off mentor for the final placement will have received specific educational preparation as determined by the NMC (2008a, 2010b), and is required to utilise a minimum of one hour a week protected time with the student in addition to the 40 per cent of placement time that they are expected to work with the mentee.

The purpose of these minimum student contact hours is to facilitate the student's learning, and assess them on the competencies that they are required to achieve during the placement, through review of requirements in the OAR document. The practice competencies booklet might have a section where the protected one hour per week is recorded, and the sign-off mentor may also ask to view the student's practice competencies booklets from all preceding place-ments, and any other skill achievement document that could contribute to the sign-off mentor's decision regarding the student's achievement of competencies.

## Signing-off proficiency

For several reasons such as ensuring validity and reliability of assessments, fair-ness of assessments, and for safe and effective practice, the assessment of compe-tence including signing-off proficiency during the final practice placement, needs to be performed by a mentor who is on the same part or sub-part of the NMC's professional register as that which the student is aiming to enter (e.g. NMC, 2009d). The NMC refers to this requirement as 'applying due regard'.

The NMC (2008a: 6–7) indicates that the 'role of the sign-off mentor is to make judgments about whether a student has achieved the required standards of proficiency for safe and effective practice for entry to the NMC register', and sign the relevant local documentation indicating that they have been achieved. When all evidence has become available to indicate that the student has successfully completed all theory and practice requirements, then the HEI informs the NMC accordingly, leading to the student applying to have their name entered on the NMC register as RN.

Signing-off proficiency is required for:

- Pre-registration nurse education programmes
- Pre-registration midwifery education programmes
- Post-registration specialist practice programmes
- SCPHNs courses.

The NMC (2010b: 1) provides further advice on the options available to enable prospective sign-off mentors to achieve sign-off mentor status, indicating that the mentor has to be supervised on at least three occasions for signing-off proficiency: the first and second occasions can be realised using a range of methods such as simulation, e-learning and OSCE, and could be achieved as part of the local NMC approved mentor preparation programme.

Signing-off proficiency is also a role that can be fulfilled by practice teachers and NMC recognised teachers, but only if they have undertaken the additional educational preparation indicated by the NMC (2008a); and they will also be required to undergo a period of precepteeship (NMC, 2007b).

Signing-off proficiency amounts to vouching for the individual's 'fitness for practice', and is therefore a role that has to be performed responsibly and accountably. However, Andrews et al. (2010) suggest that there can be problematic aspects to this role. For instance, how will inter-mentor consistency (reliability of assessments – discussed later in this chapter and in Chapter 7) be monitored? This question seems to imply that there should be a panel or peer group who can peer review the consistency and accountability of the sign-off mentor, although the designated PEF can monitor this to some extent.

Protected time for sign-off mentoring, which is one hour per week in addition to the 40 per cent of time that the student and mentor should work on the same shift, can itself be difficult to achieve in some very busy practice settings or during particularly busy periods. Furthermore, if a student is awarded a fail on this final placement, then this can raise questions about the quality of mentoring and assessment of competence that the student has experienced over the preceding two-and-a-half years of their education programme.

### Essential skills clusters

The NMC Circular 07/2007 (NMC, 2007c: 1) indicates that 'Essential skills clusters' (ESC) are 'UK-wide generic skills statements set out under broad headings that identify skills to support the achievement of the existing NMC outcomes for entry to the branch, and the proficiencies for entry to the register'. The concept emerged from the NMC consultation on pre-registration nurse education entitled *Review of Fitness for Practice at the Point of Registration* (NMC, 2006b). Respondents to the consultation were strongly in favour of ESCs, hence publication of the above-mentioned NMC Circular that details the actual skills that students must demonstrate competence in to be permitted to register as a nurse. Competence in ESCs has been a mandatory requirement for students who commenced nurse education programmes since September 2008.

Although the above-mentioned circular, as with most other NMC circulars, is subject to periodic review, it does provide guidance on the nature and implementation of ESCs. However, the five clusters of skills are reproduced in the NMC (2010a) standards of pre-registration education document, and the NMC indicates that these skills have to be incorporated at different points in education programmes based on the 2010 standards. The five clusters under which the skills are identified are:

- Care and compassion, communication
- Organisational aspects of care
- Infection prevention and control
- Nutrition and fluid management
- Medicines management.

For midwifery programmes, ESCs are also incorporated into the NMC (2009e) pre-registration midwifery education competencies, and the five ESC areas under which the skills are identified are:

1   Communication
2   Initial consultation between the woman and the midwife
3   Normal labour and birth
4   Initiation and continuance of breastfeeding
5   Medical products management.

For nursing, generic and field-specific ESC skills should be addressed within the context of each of the four fields of practice. Consequently, universities and their partner trusts design separate ESCs to be achieved by each progression point, and they are mapped against the field competencies identified by the NMC (2010a), or NMC (2009e) for midwifery education.

## Assessing AHPs, support workers, assistant practitioners

The mentor periodically gets allocated mentees who are students or learners on other health or social care profession programmes. This is of course fully acceptable especially in the current day's ethos of inter-professional learning, and endeavour towards a health and social care seamless service. This is also so that the underlying principles of mentoring and supervising learning comprise core knowledge and skills that applies to all professions. However, logically they might be required to undertake further courses to do so, or to attend relevant workshops, in particular to comprehend the technicalities of their role towards learners from other specific healthcare professions.

For example, to supervise and assess support workers on NVQ courses, they would need to have successfully completed and achieved the A1 Assessor Award (previously D32 and D33). If the nurse mentor's mentee is a medical student, then they have to acquaint themselves with the competencies that the medical student has to achieve by the end of the placement.

# Validity and Reliability of Assessments

The principles of assessment constitute further key considerations that are usually referred to as attributes or essential factors. There are four attributes that are absolutely crucial in all assessments of competencies. These are validity, reliability, discrimination and practicability (or usability) of assessments.

## Validity

'Validity' is the most crucial aspect of an assessment in that it refers to the extent to which the assessment measures what it is expected to measure. A valid assessment is one that assesses the competency or learning outcome(s) it sets out to assess, and not target other competencies that might not have been learnt adequately by the learner at that point in time. The five main types of validity are content validity, predictive validity, concurrent validity, construct validity and face validity, but some of these apply more to the overall curriculum and not necessarily to assessment of competencies in practice settings.

### Content validity
'Content validity' this refers to the extent to which the assessment adequately samples the content of the curriculum. Do the assessment question and assignment guidelines assess all the learning outcomes of the curriculum? Note that for various reasons, not everything the student learns during the course can be assessed. Content validity is primarily addressed by the structure of the assessment in the endeavour to assess all module or course outcomes, and is monitored by the programme manager for the course.

### Predictive validity
The extent to which the result of assessments can predict the future performance of the student is referred to as 'predictive validity'. It is important for the mentor to determine if the student's performance during, say, a particular practical assessment, can predict how far he or she will perform to the same

standard in future situations, and also whether they can adjust the performance to different practice settings, for example from a ward setting to community care, and to different patients.

### Concurrent validity

The extent to which the assessment results correlate with those of other assessments administered at the same time is referred to as 'concurrent validity'. In other words, if two different assessments are designed to measure the same learning outcomes, then the student should do equally well in both, for example asking a student to talk through how they would perform a skill, and actually to demonstrate it.

### Construct validity

Validity that refers to the extent to which the results of the assessment are related to impressions or evidence gained from observations of the individual's behaviour with regard to their attitudes, values and intelligence (which are also known as 'psychological constructs') is referred to as 'construct validity'.

### Face validity

'Face validity' involves stopping to consider the overall impression about how competently the clinical skill was performed, and whether the student actually demonstrates the complex array of observational, analytical, interpersonal and technical skills required for the competency.

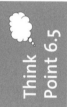

**Think Point 6.5**

## Types of validity

A first-year student is being assessed on a surgical ward changing a patient's dressing using aseptic technique. The purpose of this particular episode of assessment is specifically with regards to changing a dressing using aseptic technique skills. However, during the procedure, the patient makes some statements that clearly reflect marked disorientation, and the student is unable to respond therapeutically to disorientation. The aseptic technique is performed correctly. Should the mentor pass or fail the student? Which decision is the valid decision?

## Reliability

In addition to validity, another key consideration of any assessment is its 'reliability,' which is a term that is used to indicate the consistency with which an assessment measures what it is designed to measure. This means that if the assessment is conducted again, the same level of performance should produce the same result, provided other variables remain similar.

To take this a step further, reliability has to do with consistency in the grade or result awarded for a particular piece of work:

(a) between different mentors;
(b) between different occasions on which the work is done; and
(c) between different methods of assessment.

In all cases, the result or grades awarded should be almost or preferably exactly the same for the test to be deemed 'reliable'. Mott MacDonald (2009), the NMC's quality assurance agent, indicates that programme providers should supply evidence of systems for ensuring 'inter-rater' (referred to as 'inter-mentor' in this book) reliability and validity of assessment of competence between mentors, and measures to monitor inter-mentor reliability and validity of practice assessments.

## Reliability of assessments

Think about assessments you or your colleagues have been involved in recently. Then spend a few minutes thinking about how reliably the assessment was conducted. Decide why you think the assessment was or was not reliable.

**Think Point 6.6**

Generally, there are certain factors that might negatively affect reliability being achieved. These are practical issues such as:

- individual biases;
- halo effect;
- insufficient time allocated for the assessment;
- ambiguity of questions being asked;
- competence as an assessor;
- whether more than one assessor was involved, as two assessors could mean less subjectivity;
- whether the performance criteria had been agreed.

## Discrimination

Discrimination in assessment refers to the ability of assessment to differentiate between different levels of competence demonstrated by students, such as Year 1, Year 2 or Year 3 students. Steinaker and Bell's (1979) taxonomy of learning is generally used to differentiate between these levels of competences.

However, by and large, learners should be given the opportunity to demonstrate their true level of ability, regardless of the level he/she is expected to reach at the particular stage of the course.

Discrimination also refers to the distinction between all learners. A healthcare assistant would be assessed against different criteria for a particular clinical skill, from a medical student or from a student nurse, for instance, mainly because the level of theoretical knowledge expected of each is different.

### Practicability (or usability)

The concept 'practicability' refers to whether the assessment can be conducted within the time, and with the resources, available.

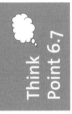

## Practicability of assessments

Think about your own practice setting. Have you encountered situations when you are required to assess a learner's competencies but felt that the time allocated was not adequate or that it was not practical to conduct the assessment comprehensively?

Mentors encounter problems of practicability of assessment when practice placements are too short, or when for some reason the assessments have been left until the last few days of the placement. In the study of assessment of competence by Phillips et al. (2000) several problems of practicability of assessment were identified, the more crucial ones of which will be explored in Chapter 7. However, despite effective assessments being complex and challenging, the validity and reliability of assessments remain the benchmark of rigour in the assessment of health and social care competencies (e.g. Rowntree, 1987; Wilkinson, 1999).

A study conducted by Norman et al. (2002: 143) that examined the validity and reliability of different methods of assessment of competence of pre-registration nursing and midwifery students, concluded that 'no single method is appropriate for assessing all clinical competence of nursing and midwifery students', and that a 'multi-method approach' should be taken.

## Implementing Approved Assessment Procedures

Each university identifies clearly in their course documents exactly which assessments students have to pass to complete the course successfully. This is supported by further assessment guidelines and specifications on how students are to acquire the necessary knowledge and competence to do so. Examples of course assessments were cited at the beginning of this chapter in response to Activity 6.1.

The procedure for assessing practice competencies is detailed in students' placement booklets. These procedures, alongside other requirements for the course will have been planned before the course starts, under the scrutiny of the university's quality assurance guidelines and protocols for designing courses and modules. Thereafter, they will have gone through a rigorous course approval process before being offered to students.

The pass marks for assessments may vary by a few points between different universities, as may the weightings between practical and theoretical assessments, or different assessment components. The number of assessments may vary, as may the number of formative assessments related to the summative ones. Each course and module is assessed on its learning outcomes, indicative content and competencies.

All universities are governed by identified boards and committees for addressing specifically designated functions related to the courses they offer. An example of a university-level board is the Academic Board and that of a committee is the Deferral Committee. Those at faculty, school or department level include the Board of Study and the Subject Assessment Board.

The functions of each of these committees – whose membership includes clinical managers, the subject librarian, the placement manager, for instance – and boards, are identified in their terms of reference. The Faculty's Board of Study for pre-registration courses, for instance, holds meetings each term to receive module and programme results, module and practice placement evaluations and issues raised at course consultative committee meetings. The mentor is not required to know in detail what each committee does, unless they are members of those committees, but some of the decisions made by these committees may affect mentoring activities with students during practice placement, such as extending the placement.

The university's Board of Study fulfils essential functions, in that it assumes ultimate responsibility for the effective delivery, evaluation and revision of modules, courses and the students' programmes of studies, some of the feedback for which it receives from relevant Faculty Board(s). It tends to have an overall monitoring role in relation to module or course assessments. During the planning stages, the modules will have been fully discussed by the Course or Module Curriculum Planning Teams. They will have been designed following the university's protocol. It would, for instance, have followed the university's protocol for writing modules, and the university's Assessment Parity Rules, which include rules on word limits for coursework. They would then have been approved by an assembled panel of experts, which usually includes representations from the NMC, probably the HPC, and subject specialists from other universities.

Furthermore, in addition to the overall university assessment strategy there are specific assessment strategies within each course and module, thereby ensuring that each programme is fully structured before students start on the course.

## Policies and strategies for assessments

For assessment of practice, students' practice placement competencies booklets clearly identify the procedure for assessment of competencies. This entails an initial mentor–mentee interview when the competencies to be achieved are ascertained, and often a learning contract constituted. Approximately halfway through the placement a mid-placement interview takes place to ascertain the student's progress with the contracted competencies. During the last week of the placement a final interview is conducted for the decision on which clinical competencies have been achieved, and those that have are signed and dated accordingly.

To do so, various strategies are advocated for assessment of clinical skills, such as direct observation of skill performance, writing a reflective account, questions and answers, etc. It is usually up to the mentor to decide which NMC competency area can be assessed by each strategy. For example, direct observation can be utilised for assessing clinical skill, attitude, communication skill; and questions and answers for the rationale for each action taken, knowledge of the effects of medication, etc.

A variety or 'diversity' of assessment strategies is also recommended by the QAA (2006) to enable students to demonstrate their capabilities and achievements of module or programme outcomes; and by the NMC (2010a). For assessment of theory components, critical analyses of key concepts and seminar presentations, written examinations are utilised. It is, however, well known that some assessment methods, e.g. written examinations, enable some students to demonstrate their capabilities more effectively, whilst other methods suit other students better. Garside et al. (2009) explored the feasibility and outcome of allowing students a choice of assessment methods, and found that this is achievable, as some students chose to be assessed by seminar discussions, others by poster presentations, others by essays, etc., to good effect.

Consequently, curriculum planners should be able to justify which modes of assessment tests which module or programme outcome more effectively, and complementarily the NMC (2008a) indicates that mentors should also be able to demonstrate understanding and ability to utilise a range of assessment strategies. Research on the effective use of assessment strategies is scarce.

However, in a study that explored the extent to which mentors use different assessment strategies in Ireland, McCarthy and Murphy (2008) found that a limited range of these were in use. McCarthy and Murphy recommend further research on utilisation of assessment strategies, and further education of mentors on their use.

All aforementioned proceedings are documented as evidence of progress with continuous assessment, for the final summative assessment of the practice module, and for legal reasons. The practice competencies' booklets also identify the exact roles and responsibilities of the mentor, those of the student before, during and after the placement. They also contain a set of components related to the student's professionalism, attitude and their teamworking, and which the student must demonstrate at a satisfactory level (related to construct validity). Usually there is also a section on actions to take regarding under-achieving students, which is explored in Chapter 7.

## Chapter Summary

This chapter has focused on the assessment of learner's clinical knowledge and competences, taking the approach of what are assessments, why do we conduct them, who assesses, when and how, which encompassed:

- What the term 'assessment' means, in the context of assessing professional knowledge and competence. This involved considering various definitions of assessments, and the exact competencies to be assessed.
- Why we need to assess our students and learners, that is the exact purposes and aims of assessments, and at which particular points in students' programmes of study to assess.
- Who assesses learners, including student self-assessment, and peer assessment, and patient or service user involvement in assessment of competencies.
- How assessments are conducted, which includes ensuring the mentee has learned the clinical skill, the use of essential interpersonal skills, the dimensions of assessments, namely continuous or episodic assessments, formative or summative and criterion-referenced or norm-referenced assessments.
- Assessing different levels of competence, fairness of assessments and the use of performance criteria.
- Validity, reliability, discrimination and practicability as essential aspects of assessments; and the role of approved assessment policies, procedures and strategies.

## Further Optional Reading

For an analysis of problematic aspects of assessment, the danger of which recurring usually looms, see:

- Rowntree, D. (1987) *Assessing Students: How Shall We Know Them?* London: Kogan Page.

Print *Standards for Pre-registration Nurse Education* or *Standards of Proficiency* documents from the NMC or HPC internet website, either to gain an overview, or for more detailed scrutiny of the standards and outcomes that preregistration students have to achieve to be able to register in the relevant part of the Professional Register.

- Nursing and Midwifery Council (2010a) *Standards for Pre-registration Nursing Education.* Available at: http://standards.nmc-uk.org/PreRegNursing/statutory/background/Pages/Introduction.aspx. Accessed 18 September 2010.

For specific up-to-date procedures for clinical interventions in adult nursing (there are similar but not identical textbooks for other fields of practice such as mental health nursing), see:

- Dougherty, L. and Lister, S. (eds) (2008) *The Royal Marsden Hospital Manual of Clinical Nursing Procedures* (8th edn). Oxford: Blackwell.

For more detailed information on criteria and processes for achieving sign-off mentor status, see Sections 2.1.3 and 3.2.6 of:

- Nursing and Midwifery Council (2008a) *A Standard to Support Learning and Assessment in Practice.* London: NMC.

For an in-depth analysis of how to implement a new assessment strategy, in this case concept mapping (with poster presentation and discussion), see:

- Akinsanya, C. and Williams, M. (2004) 'Concept mapping for meaningful learning', *Nurse Education Today*, 24 (1): 41–6.

For further details of actions that mentors should take in different situations and at critical points during mentoring, presented as bullet points lists, see:

- Royal College of Nursing (2007) *Guidance for Mentors of Nursing Students and Midwives: An RCN Toolkit.* London: RCN.

# 7
# Leadership and the Challenges of Mentoring

## Introduction

Mentors are generally informed of the student allocated to them well before the practice placement starts, to which the mentor responds by structuring a tentative plan of learning experiences for the learner for the duration of the placement. Research findings (e.g. Phillips et al., 2000; Duffy, 2003; Gainsbury, 2010) highlight various day-to-day problems that could be encountered by both mentors and students in the assessment of students' competencies during practice placements. That assessments are conducted 'on the hoof' by registrants the assessee 'bumps into', and as part of 'multiple roles', were issues highlighted by Phillips et al. (2000); 'failure to fail' was the main problem highlighted by Duffy (2003), as well as by Gainsbury (2010) as sometimes mentors award a pass to students without sufficient evidence of their competence in specific clinical skills. Similarly, O'Driscoll et al. (2010) identify problems with mentoring such as workload interfering with facilitation of students' learning during practice placements, and mentors feeling pressurised to take on the mentor role for their career development.

Such problems can fully or partly be averted by the mentor's leadership, which includes accepting the role as a serious responsibility, and early forward planning. The NMC (2008a: 58), under the leadership domain, indicates that mentors should 'Demonstrate leadership skills for education within practice and academic settings', the associated outcomes for which are:

- plan a series of learning experiences that will meet students' defined learning needs;
- be an advocate for students to support them accessing learning opportunities that meet their individual needs, involving a range of other professionals, patients, clients and carers;
- prioritise work to accommodate support of students within their practice roles;
- provide feedback about the effectiveness of learning and assessment in practice.

These outcomes reflect the mentor's leadership in the context of planning for the placement, prioritising, supporting and giving feedback. As for planning 'learning experiences' and 'accessing learning opportunities', these components were discussed in Chapter 1 to a good extent, and in Chapter 4 in more detail. Careful forward planning of own work and prioritising are key features of the mentor's leadership role towards achievement of placement competencies, as is acting proactively to avert the likely contemporary problems of assessments, and dealing with those that do occur. At the end of the placement, the mentor has to inform the student of their levels of achievement, and of a decision to award the student a pass or fail for those assessment components. It is in relation to assessment of competence that mentors encounter most of the challenges to their role.

## Chapter outcomes

On completion of this chapter, you should be able to:

1  Explain specific ways in which forward planning and prioritising work comprise important means by which the mentor exercises leadership.
2  Identify likely problems of assessment of competencies, and ways in which the mentor averts or resolves them.
3  Present an analysis of the responsibilities and accountability of the mentor in the assessment of practice competencies, along with related ethical and legal aspects of mentoring.
4  Ascertain ways in which the mentor achieves and monitors intra- and inter-mentor reliability in the decisions they make in relation to the assessments they conduct.
5  Ascertain the mentor's role in supporting the struggling or under-achieving student, and the use of various lines of support that can be available to them, including resources and guidelines.

## The Mentor's Leadership in Managing Assessments

The mentor's leadership related to pre-registration and post-qualifying education in healthcare professions has been identified by research for some time (e.g. Fretwell, 1980; Phillips et al., 2000; O'Driscoll et al., 2010).

According to O'Driscoll and colleagues, personnel who are in a position to take the lead include clinical nurse specialists, modern matrons, nurse consultants, nurse practitioners, nurse managers, and others of similar seniority, but their role in student teaching during practice placements is less well defined. They also found, however, that the ward manager's leadership in creating an environment for learning in the practice setting is crucial, and also that it is the mentor who exercises leadership in facilitation of learning more regularly and fully.

Leadership as a notion in its own right was referred to in Chapter 5 in the context of healthcare professionals acting as change agents in the management of change (see Table 5.2 for the approaches taken by transactional and transformational leaders). There are several definitions of leadership prevalent in management literature, most of which emphasise the leader's ability to *influence* the activities, behaviour or actions of their 'followers' towards goal achievement. In the context of healthcare, Gopee and Galloway (2009: 48) suggest that 'leadership comprises the ability to motivate, inspire and energise individuals and groups to identify and achieve healthcare goals'. These abilities also apply to effective mentoring.

Leadership skills are also a feature recommended for preceptee programmes, which the NMC is considering making a mandatory requirement as part of the most recently reviewed pre-registration nurse education standards published in 2010. Other areas that the newly qualified nurse will develop as part of their precepteeship are clinical, research and teaching skills. For a thorough and up-to-date analysis of leadership as a concept that applies to most areas of society, the reader is referred to Kouzes and Posner's (2007) *The Leadership Challenge*.

Assessment of competencies at times involves one-off short episodes of direct observation of the learner performing clinical skills in accordance with the trust's procedure. Otherwise, it is a continual process occurring throughout the practice placement. Assessment of theory is conducted and managed by the university through coursework essays and written examinations, but the process of assessment of students' competencies has to be managed by the mentor.

The various problems that are likely to be associated with assessments make early and careful planning of assessment imperative. Such planning constitutes an endeavour to ensure that the learner achieves the identified learning objectives for the placement, and to pre-empt problems. There is also the danger that if interruptions do occur during episodes of assessment, then the mentor could miss vital steps in the performance of the skill and decide on a pass (or fail) with insufficient information. Incorrect or unsafe practice can be missed.

## Managing the process of assessment in the practice setting

---

### Activity 7.1   Planning and managing the process of assessment of practice

This activity asks you to explore in detail how to manage the assessment of students' competencies or clinical skills. To do this, focus on the specified outcomes or competencies of a specific practice module of the pre-registration course for your healthcare profession, or the NMC's (2010a) competencies for, say, second year students in your field of nursing, or the outcomes of a post-registration healthcare course. Practice module outcomes are normally found in the student's practice competencies or outcomes booklet.

You might choose to work with a colleague or course peer who is in a similar specialism as you on this activity. Identify in detail everything that needs to be done to begin and complete the assessment of these competencies, from the time the student starts on the practice placement to when the student is signed as competent for particular competencies. Include everything such as how you'd ensure the skills (or knowledge/attitude) have been learnt, and organisational aspects that have to be considered to ensure the assessment proceeds as planned.

---

From your response to Activity 7.1, you would have verbalised various preparations needed to ensure assessment of competencies is completed effectively and efficiently. Maybe the mentor can compile a teaching and assessment schedule that identifies which competencies will have been learnt by the student by the end of week two, three, etc., and at which points the mentor will have assessed the student on each of them, as also suggested broadly by Price (2007). The learning and assessment schedule of course needs to be flexible enough to allow for opportunistic or incidental learning, otherwise it needs to be adhered to as planned, and can form part of a 'learning agreement' (as explained in Chapter 1).

For all assessments there are usually certain curriculum regulations that need to be adhered to, such as submission dates for practice competencies booklets, and the procedure to follow if the student fails a competency. A number of key points specifically related to managing practical assessments are identified in Box 7.1.

## Box 7.1    Planning and managing the assessment process

**In sequence**

| | |
|---|---|
| Prior to the assessment | • Agree, during week 1 of placement, the objectives/competencies that need to be achieved and assessed. |
| | • Ensure that the learner has learnt the skill, allocate registrants to teach the skill in accordance with agreed performance criteria. The skill is taught at the appropriate academic level. The learner is given sufficient practice opportunities and has been formatively assessed during the placement. |
| | • Mentor feels: (a) up to date with skills being assessed; (b) competent to assess/has attended mentor update course; (c) takes a supportive and positive approach. |
| | • Day of assessment – ensure that the student feels ready for the assessment, set time of day, consider 'practicability' and fairness of assessment issues. |
| | • Colleagues aware if and when they can interrupt (if necessary), give bleep/pager to another person. |
| | • Agree performance criteria. |
| During the assessment | • Use appropriate communication skills (see Box 6.1). |
| | • Create a climate that enables the student to relax so that they can perform the skill to the best of their ability. |
| | • Safety issues – if assessee makes a mistake, consider seriousness of mistake, and intervene, or provide prompt/clues, as appropriate. |
| | • Responsive assessment (Neary, 2000b) – taking into account the patient's changing healthcare needs. |
| | • Situated assessments, i.e. in the context of available resources, and clinical activities, for instance. |
| | • Consider predictive validity of assessments, i.e. whether the assessee can perform as well in future and in other patient care situations. |
| After the assessment | • Need to exercise professional judgement throughout. |
| | • Decide on whether to award a pass or fail for each skill or competency assessed. |

*(Continued)*

*(Continued)*

- Give feedback according to established good practice (discussed next).
- Ensure documentation is complete – for clinical intervention, student competency, and of feedback given.
- If fail is awarded, then the mentor needs to follow the university's procedure for subsequent actions to take, which normally includes informing the link tutor or the PEF.

## Making decisions and giving feedback to the assessee

Following assessment of competency, the mentor has to indicate to the assessee whether they have passed or failed. Prior to this, however, the mentor needs to give feedback to the assessee on their performance of the clinical skill because all assessments should be learning situations, and the feedback should motivate the assessee to reflect on how to improve performance, or build on a good performance. Feedback is also a means of justifying the pass or fail result. Feedback can be: (a) *intrinsic feedback*, which occurs within the performer through self-assessment and reflection (the student often knows how well or not so well they did); or (b) *extrinsic feedback* (or augmented feedback), which is given by the assessor or peers and done concurrently during the skill performance, and/or on completion of the performance. Some mentors find it difficult to give honest feedback on a weak or faulty student performance. This could be tricky for the assessee as well, but feedback has to be given honestly, and is generally accepted more readily if given constructively.

It is useful to ask the assessee how they felt they performed straight (or soon) after completion of the clinical skill, instead of telling them first how well or badly they performed. The benefits of asking the student are that this is likely to make them put aside any anxiety they might still have about their performance, think more objectively, and be more receptive to feedback. So, the mentor could ask, 'How do you think you did?' This constitutes self-assessment by the learner (which was discussed in Chapter 6), which should also give the mentor an indication of the learner's insights into their level of competence. Good practice guidelines for giving feedback to students are listed in Box 7.2.

## Box 7.2   Guidelines for giving feedback to the student after clinical skill performance

- Ensure privacy, and that adequate time is allocated.
- Use the sandwich method, which entails starting with comments on the positive points or strengths, discussing areas for improvement, and ending on positive notes.
- Give feedback constructively, as the aim of feedback is to enable the learner to learn and improve.
- Be sensitive to the recipient's feelings and self-esteem throughout this exercise.
- Try to be honest and fair but never be destructive.
- Be clear and concise.
- Allow the recipient of the feedback time to discuss and ask for clarification.
- Do not allow anxiety levels to increase unduly.
- Gauge the impact of your feedback on the student's feelings and self-esteem throughout the exercise.
- Respect and treat the recipient as an individual, and focus upon behaviour and skill performance rather than personality traits (i.e. mustn't be perceived as a personal remark).
- Acknowledge good practice.
- Suggest measures to correct inappropriate practice.
- Remain calm and objective; do not respond in kind to anger, aggression and defensiveness.
- Motivate the recipient to consolidate strengths and address limitations through strategies such as action plans.
- Be empowering through encouragement of the recipient to comment and explain issues discussed.

Good general communication skills are essential when giving feedback, including non-verbal communication such as maintaining eye contact. Following feedback, action plans or learning points can be constituted and mutually agreed, as also suggested by the RCN (2007). However, in an ethos of self-directed learning, ultimately it is up to the receiver of the feedback to decide how much of it to heed and act upon, and when, and to be accountable for their decisions.

## Good practice guidelines for assessments

This section builds on the important principles of assessment of clinical skills performance discussed in Chapter 6, and in some current literature such as

DH (2001b) and Rowntree (1987). A set of guidelines for the day-to-day mechanics of assessment is therefore constituted and presented in Box 7.3.

---

## Box 7.3    Good practice guidelines for the day-to-day mechanics of assessment

- Allocate mentors for teaching specific skill/knowledge
- Utilise opportunities for formative assessments
- Arrange time and date, and diary it; treat it as 'protected time' (e.g. DH, 1999; NMC, 2008a)
- Inform other staff to ensure they do not interrupt (considering staffing levels of course)
- Inform patient and obtain permission for student assessment
- Ensure all equipment is available
- Ensure assessee has had opportunity to practise the skill
- Ensure mentor is fully available and accessible
- Be sensitive to the student's self-confidence or lack of it
- Be aware of any crises in the practice setting, e.g. staff sickness, stress
- Plan the assessment, ensuring availability of procedures and guidelines
- Take safety measures if required
- Work in teams as this strengthens the reliability of assessments
- Seek the opinions of colleagues who have experience of working with the learner being assessed, when feasible
- Create opportunity for learner to talk through the procedure, if necessary
- Always remain calm
- If the assessee displays awe of the assessor, give confidence
- Beware of unachievable goals
- Be and look enthusiastic and motivated
- Allow student to work at their own pace
- Allow for holistic care
- Ensure assessee knows the performance criteria for the skill
- Allow reflection and give feedback
- Use professional judgement
- Beware of other factors, e.g. learner being preoccupied with assignments
- Heed criticisms of assessments, e.g. research findings such as 'failing to fail' (Duffy, 2003), and 'on-the-hoof' assessments (Phillips et al., 2000)
- Intervene appropriately if unsafe practice is about to occur
- Do not be biased by occasional polarised instances of exceptionally thorough or poor practice
- Document results as required by the assessment strategy

Various viewpoints discussed so far suggest that appropriate documentation is vital to mentoring activities. In fact, documentation of assessments is crucial, considering the NMC's (2009c) position that recording comprises documentary evidence of actions taken.

---

## Activity 7.2   The student's practice competencies

Look through your copy (mentor's copy) or the student's copy of the practice competencies booklet, and read the sections where it identifies the roles of the mentor, the link tutor and personal tutor, and of the student during the placement.

---

A clause in the booklet usually states the actions that the mentor needs to take if the mentee is perceived as underachieving or 'failing'. They tend to entail drawing on the expertise of mentor colleagues, the link tutor, the PEF or the student's personal tutor. There is also usually a section on the appeals procedure. However, for each new course or module being offered, there would have been a briefing session for prospective mentors to familiarise themselves with the course requirements, the specific competencies to be achieved by students, and to discuss issues.

If you are on a mentoring course yourself, it is very important that, on completion of the course, before you conduct any student assessment, you acquaint yourself with the student's placement competencies, and preferably the overall assessment strategy for the course. Furthermore, you should fully understand the particular summative assessment that you are going to conduct. The action to take in case of 'failure to achieve required standard' by the learner, and the 'appeals procedure' are discussed later in this chapter. The importance of careful forward planning to ensure assessments of practice competencies proceed systematically during practice placement, to prevent problems surfacing, to maximise learning, and to reduce the likelihood of the student experiencing undue stress, are all extremely important.

The NMC (2008a) recommends that mentors and their managers should endeavour to quantify and allocate 'protected time' for mentoring. Despite careful planning, unfolding day-to-day events could still disrupt the smooth running of assessments. The patient could refuse consent to students performing skills on them, staff sickness, unexpected emergency admissions or referrals might present as obstacles. However, these do not always present as problems, as Neary (2000a), Philips et al. (2000), and others recommend 'responsive assessment', which entails taking into account situational contexts such as prevailing resource issues, and the patient's current physiological or psychological state.

### Intra- and inter-mentor reliability

Mentor preparation courses usually also incorporate an exploration of how intra- and inter-mentor reliability are achieved and monitored after qualifying as a mentor, especially in relation to conducting assessments, which has also been identified as an essential mentor activity previously by the NMC's predecessor organisations.

Mott MacDonald (2009), the NMC's quality assurance agent, refers to these as intra- and inter-rater reliability. Rating, in the context of assessment of competencies, refers to the mentor deciding on the quality (see Niklin and Kenworthy's (2000) definition of assessment in Chapter 6) of the student's performance or response to their teaching. The quality of student performance in practice competencies is even graded (e.g. between A and F) in some HEI courses where the mechanism has been instituted, and the necessary educational preparation delivered.

The term *intra-mentor reliability*, in the mentor's assessment role, refers to how consistently the mentor assesses particular categories of students on particular clinical skills, that is, that he or she consistently uses the same identified performance criteria for a skill, within a responsive assessment approach. *Inter-mentor reliability* refers to the consistency with which all mentors assess a particular category of students on particular clinical skills.

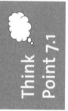

**Think Point 7.1**

## Intra- and inter-mentor reliability

Think of ways in which mentors can achieve and monitor intra- and inter-mentor reliability. What are the informal and more structured situations or opportunities that they can utilise to explore these?

As you would have sensed, intra- and inter-mentor reliability refer to all roles of the mentor, such as those enunciated in the eight NMC (2008a) domains, associated competences and outcomes for the mentor, although it is usually related to assessments. There are various ways of monitoring intra- and inter-mentor reliability. One of the most effective of these is through discussion groups or workshops on mentor update study days. All mentors are required to attend annual updates to remain on the university's or trusts' local register (or database) of current mentors (NMC, 2008a). The update study days and trust-based mentor update sessions provide a suitable opportunity to raise any issues and also to explore consistency within and across mentors. Case studies can be examined in small groups, or these groups can be invited to discuss consistency in the context of situations they've personally encountered as mentors. In these groups, conclusions can be drawn on consistency in assessments conducted by mentors, and with the help of the facilitator, benchmarks of good practice can be established.

However, monitoring intra- and inter-mentor reliability mustn't wait for update study days. Informal monitoring is undertaken continuously through discussions with peers or team members in the practice setting or unit, with one's line manager, or the mentor's own mentor or clinical supervisor.

Further ways of achieving intra-mentor reliability are by:

- Consistently using approved protocols/clinical guidelines.
- Ascertaining that approved procedures and clinical guidelines are up to date.
- Ensuring own competence and skills are up to date.
- Informal monitoring of own pass/fail rates of mentees.
- Ensuring appropriate environment for assessing, for example, the transferability of competence from skills laboratories to different care settings (i.e. community, critical care).
- Ensuring that the learner is being taught to the same standard and protocol/procedure by different registrants/associate mentors.
- Student feedback such as evaluating how the student feels about the assessment process and decisions.
- External feedback, from colleagues through reflections on assessments conducted.
- Ensuring that learners are aware of level of performance expected of them.
- Reflection-on-action on assessment just conducted.
- Ensuring being aware of halo effect, being non-judgemental, for instance about the assessee as a person; objectivity.
- Being consistent in own standard of clinical practice.

In addition to the above-mentioned ways of achieving reliability of assessments, inter-mentor reliability is achieved by:

- Mentor meetings within ward/unit team – formal and informal.
- Involving PEF when uncertain.
- Consulting colleagues on same ward/unit as appropriate.
- Auditing mentor's performance of assessments (e.g. by negotiating peer assessment).
- Student feedback about mentoring practices.
- Feedback from university following student evaluations.
- Monitoring attendance at mentor updates, trust-based or university-based.
- Knowing and consulting/informing link tutor.
- Exploring mentoring issues at clinical supervision meetings.
- Ensuring same clinical guidelines/protocols were being used.
- Monitoring mentors are up to date with clinical skills.

# Averting and Resolving Problems of Assessments

Potential problems of assessment of practice competencies can be averted by careful planning, and this is the component wherein the mentor's leadership is absolutely essential. However, problems with assessments do occur and, when they do, they have to be treated as a component of mentoring, and resolved, and efforts made to learn from them.

## Potential problems of assessment of competence

The aims or purposes of assessments are quite clearly identified by several writers on nurse education, as noted under 'Why do we need to assess our students?' in Chapter 6. However, how far and how smoothly these aims are achieved in reality varies. We also need to consider exactly what the problems that mentors encounter in the assessment of students are, and what the criticisms directed at assessments are, including those of written examinations.

---

### Activity 7.3   Current problems of assessments

Think of the weaknesses of assessments and reasons why assessments, even written examinations, are unpopular with students (assuming they are). Make brief notes.

Identify the actual problems that tend to occur with student assessment of theory and practice in your healthcare profession, ones that you have experienced or observed, or that you feel could occur.

---

Mentors and learners could encounter various difficulties with assessment of practice competencies. For assessment of theoretical knowledge (e.g. of human physiology) and numerical skills as in drug administration and nurse prescribing courses, written examinations remain a favoured method, particularly in higher education. The likely solutions to the problems that you have identified will be explored shortly. A range of problems of assessments was identified by just one group of students on a mentoring course. These are presented in Box 7.4.

---

### Box 7.4   Problems with assessments

- Leaving things to the last minute (i.e. poor time planning)
- Difficulty with integration of theory and practice, or ineffective application

*(Continued)*

*(Continued)*
- Personality problems/clashes
- Problems of organisation in the practice setting
- Lack of time
- Student disagrees with mentor
- Attitude problems – student's or mentor's
- Structure of learning programme (e.g. placement is too short)
- Mentor accountable and responsible for how student performs the clinical intervention
- Inconsistency of student performance
- Student absence
- Mentor low morale
- Mentor changes or absence
- Student appears indifferent
- Student's level of knowledge
- Lack of resources (e.g. equipment)
- Non-cooperation or refusal of consent by the patient or service user

One of the most cited difficulties mentors face is insufficient time for mentoring activities. Cognisance of this recurrent problem necessitates more robust leadership on the part of the mentor in terms of forward planning, prioritising and proactive actions. The substantial empirical study on assessments by Phillips et al. (2000) highlighted various problems encountered by assessors, which are:

1  The quality of assessment varies enormously, depending on staffing levels and workload in the practice setting.
2  Named assessors perform their assessor role as one of many other essential roles.
3  Many assessments are performed informally by registrants the assessee 'bumps into' during the course of their duty (i.e. 'opportunistic' and 'piecemeal').
4  Few assessment schedules recognise theories derived from day-to-day 'real' clinical practice, and remain a problem for assessors.
5  A major part of registrants' practice involves solving the operational and ethical dilemmas they regularly face in 'situations' with competing demands on their time.
6  The most valid assessments are those of: (a) 'situated understanding' (explained under 8); and (b) judgement that occurs as a result of close observation of the assessee over a sustained period by the assessor.
7  Nursing and midwifery practice has to meet the expectations of a wide range of stakeholders, including individual patients and relatives, individual practitioners, user groups, Trusts, HEIs, SHAs, the healthcare professions regulatory bodies and the Department of Health.
8  The conditions under which assessees are assessed are variable but should always be 'situated' and therefore take into account the constraints and possibilities in the practice setting.

9   Mentors experience difficulty in ascertaining different levels in practice.
10   Few assessors feel well prepared for doing assessments and most express a desire for continuing support after initial preparation, and consideration of adequate infrastructure for valid and reliable assessments.

In more general terms, an earlier study conducted by Satterly (1981) high-lighted weaknesses with assessments that can still occur, and can arise across academic subjects. Satterly identified several 'objections to assessments', such as assessments being limited to achieving specific outcomes at the expense of the general aims of education. He suggested that some types of assessments constitute an invasion of privacy of the individual, that assessments encourage pupils to develop the styles of thought or intellectual 'tricks' required for passing tests, and not the skills that education would wish them to achieve.

Many of these weaknesses could occur in healthcare courses, although actions have since been taken to remedy some of them. For instance, with regards to assessments being limited to relatively trivial outcomes, a curriculum that is too focused on assessment of specific objectives could overlook some of the more important aims of education. With regards to the aims of higher education, Entwistle (1994) identifies these as:

- Adopting a distinctive way of thinking about concepts, evidence and theories.
- Taking a distanced, critical stance towards subject matter, assumptions and explanations.
- Tackling issues systematically, logically and effectively.
- Examining the adequacy of evidence and checking alternative interpretations of it.
- Demonstrating a thorough understanding of complex, abstract concepts within the discipline.
- Writing clearly and cogently, following appropriate academic styles and conventions.
- Being able to set and solve problems by applying concepts and techniques appropriately.

The QAA (2008) provides detailed aims of education for different years of study in HEIs. In university-based healthcare courses, the aims of higher education are assessed mostly in theoretical assessments, where critical analysis, problem solving and evidence of arguments presented are expected.

As for Satterly's (1981) reference to assessments as invasions of privacy of the individual, this could apply to assessment of learners in that if a learner is struggling to achieve their practice competencies for no obvious reasons, then the mentor and others may probe for personal reasons for the learner not achieving. With an increasingly mature student population, family responsibilities, single motherhood, and having to hold down part-time jobs while on the pre-registration course could well all be reasons for a student not being able to give course matters sufficient attention, and therefore not achieving. Some students can be put off by this and even drop out of the course for a better-paid vocation. Others may accept extra help.

It is also suggested that patient privacy could be invaded during assessments, in that instead of one healthcare professional performing a procedure with a patient, when student assessment is being conducted then the student and the mentor are both present. Students might also take longer to perform the procedure, and if the mentor asks the student questions during the assessment, then the procedure can be even more prolonged, with the undesirable consequence of even the patient's body part being exposed for longer periods of time. Additionally, in healthcare, invasion of privacy in assessment might also include problems of confidentiality (e.g. in reflective write-ups in patient-based assessments).

Other problems with assessments have been identified by Rowntree (1987), Nicklin and Kenworthy (2000), Lankshear (1990) and Duffy (2003). Rowntree discusses some of the 'side-effects of assessments', referring to concepts such as self-fulfilling prophecy, whereby students who are expected to achieve low grades tend to achieve low grades, which might not necessarily be a reflection of their innate ability. On the other hand, Nicklin and Kenworthy argue that the criticisms of assessments are essentially criticisms of schemes of assessment in certain curricula, or faulty implementation. The findings of Lankshear's and Duffy's studies are discussed shortly.

## Difficulties with assessment of clinical skills

### Activity 7.4    Difficulties with student assessment

Think about current day-to-day potential problems of assessments, and, considering them in the context of your own current place of work, first identify at least one clinical assessor who has already conducted quite a few clinical assessments. She or he does not need to be based solely in your workplace but should work broadly within your specialism. Your task is then to approach the assessor and ask them to explain precisely what steps they take in preparation for, and in actually conducting, assessment of competence with learners. Find out also from the assessor how they anticipate potential problems and avert them. Ask about some of the actual problems encountered, and the options they had for resolving them.

At the same time or afterwards, reflect for yourself on such problems and decide how you would go about dealing with them if they occurred in your own practice setting.

Alternatively, think for yourself of all the problems that you might encounter in your assessment function as a mentor, and then the options that will be available to you to resolve each of them.

Problems of assessment include differences in the interpretation of the exact meaning of placement objectives. There might be problems in conveying depth of knowledge expected, or level of skill demonstration. Issues like these can be rectified by open discussion between all personnel directly involved.

## Resolving problems of assessments

---

### Activity 7.5    Resolving difficulties encountered by mentors

Refer back to Box 7.4 and work on the difficulties faced by mentors by identifying a number of problems of assessment you could encounter with a particular group of students, and the probable solutions for each of them. This can be done by completing Table 7.1.

---

The chances are that you will be aware of or have thought of yet other problematic situations encountered by mentors in the assessment of learners, for which similar steps can be taken. They might include passing a student

TABLE 7.1   Criticisms or difficulties with assessments, and actions that can be taken to resolve them

| Criticisms/difficulties with assessments | Actions that can be taken to resolve them |
|---|---|
| Leaving things to the last minute | |
| Difficulty with integration, or ineffective application, of theory and practice | |
| Personality problems/clashes | |
| Problems of organisation | |
| Lack of time for conducting assessments | |
| Student disagrees with mentor | |
| Attitude problems – student's or mentor's | |
| The service user or patient not consenting to student assessment | |
| Lack of resources (e.g. equipment) | |
| Structure of learning programme: variation of experience, e.g. allocation too short | |
| ............. (other) | |

because the mentor likes the student, or failing the student because they d
like them, unqualified mentors signing up clinical competencies or misint
pretation of wording of practice competencies.

With some of these problem areas there could be instances when a mentor passes a student on a particular competency when they should be awarding a fail. This cannot be condoned, but failure to fail students has already
been identified over the years by, for example, Lankshear (1990), Duffy
(2003), and more recently by Gainsbury (2010). If a student is failing, the
mentor's professional judgement comes into play, and action plans are
constructed.

## Action planning

A mid-placement interview during the practice placement is an important
component of assessment of students' progress with their placement competencies. The competencies will have been agreed at the beginning of the placement, and might be in the form of a learning contract. The mid-placement
interview is technically a formal formative assessment point, which involves
dedicated time for a discussion on, and documentation of, the student's
progress with placement competencies.

If the student has been progressing mostly as expected, then these are
documented and the student continues as agreed in the learning contract. If
the student has not been achieving as expected in knowledge, skills and
attitudes components, then a negotiated action plan needs to be constructed,
which both mentor and learner mutually agree and sign. A PEF or an academic such as the link tutor might also be present and sign the action plan
accordingly. The important components of an action plan are presented in
Table 7.2 – it is usually laid out in landscape format.

Action planning involves specifying all components identified at the top of
the table. If such an action plan was not constituted, then the student could have
grounds for complaint and appeal if he or she is subsequently deemed a 'fail' for
the placement. This point also indicates the importance of documentation of
progress with achievement of placement objectives.

While there are some similarities between learning contracts and action
plans, there are distinct differences between them in that the former is more
learning centred and the latter is more assessment centred. The learning contract is a systematic but speculative plan of learning based on practice competencies to be achieved and projected learning opportunities, and they may
be adjusted during mid-placement progress discussions. The action plan is a
'must-achieve' device that identifies competencies that need to be achieved
by an identified date during the practice placement, non-achievement of
which would lead to a 'fail' mark being awarded.

**TABLE 7.2** Example of an action plan

| ACTION PLAN | | Mentee's name: | | | Mentor's name: |
|---|---|---|---|---|---|
| Mentee's learning needs | Specific objectives to be achieved | Who will help mentee achieve the objectives and how? | Other resources required | Achieve by dates | Evidence of achievement of objectives |
| Risk assessment for falls | Ability to assess the likelihood of an older patient falling when mobilising unaided | Mentor, physiotherapist. Support learning in actual patient or service user situations | Local criteria and clinical guidelines related to falls | 29 July 2011 | Demonstrate ability to assess accurately the risk of an older patient sustaining a fall when mobilising |
| Medicines management | Ability to administer medication safely according to local drug policy | ..... | ..... | ..... | ..... |
| ..... | | ..... | | | |

AGREEMENT OF ACTION PLAN

Mentor's signature: ................. Date: 17 June 2011 Student's signature: ................. Date: .................

ACHIEVEMENT OF OBJECTIVES

Mentor's signature: ................. Date: .................

## Re-assessing the learner

Once the action plan has been agreed, it must be adhered to, in that the mentor (or PEF) and the student jointly ensure that the competencies are being acquired, continuous assessment is occurring and, when ready, the student is reassessed and the documentation signed as and when achieved. The action plan is regularly reviewed and at the agreed date a final review is conducted.

The components discussed in the preceding section addressed mostly the duties of the mentor. The next section considers the ethical and legal aspects of mentoring.

# Ethical and Legal Aspects of Assessments

All registrants have to comply with their professional body's code of practice, and this applies to mentoring or supervising juniors' and colleagues' learning as well. 'Professional values' is one of the 'domains' of generic and field competencies that addresses ethical and legal aspects that the NMC (2010a) identifies as components that student nurses must achieve for gaining entry to the professional register. These are located under the domain 'Professional and ethical practice' in the preceding standards (NMC, 2004a).

Therefore the mentor should already be knowledgeable of legal and ethical aspects of professional practice through their pre-registration preparation, while their mentees will be developing these through theirs. On exploring the ethics of mentoring, Brown (2005) suggests that the mentor needs to be aware of their own values and ethical interpretations of clinical practice to enable mentees to develop 'ethical competence'.

Ethics refers to the social behaviours, morals and values of individuals and groups in relation to doing good for the greatest number, and to the impact or end results of clinical interventions (adapted from Brown, 2005). One widely accepted set of principles of ethics that apply to many spheres of life, including medicine, business and education, has been formulated by Thiroux and Krasemann (2007). These principles are:

- the value of life;
- goodness and rightness;
- justice and fairness;
- truth-telling and honesty;
- individual freedom.

These principles apply directly to instances of mentoring in the following way:

- *The value of life* – can refer to ensuring mentees develop the necessary competencies for effective clinical interventions that would restore health and well-being. It can also refer to ensuring mentees acquire the necessary knowledge, skills and attitudes to register as a nurse so that they can earn a livelihood.
- *Goodness and rightness* – refer to the mentor doing good to mentees and patients or service users, and doing the right things.
- *Justice and fairness* – refer to ensuring that all mentees acquire the knowledge, skills and attitudes in appropriate detail and depth.
- *Truth-telling and honesty* – ensuring incorrect information is not given.
- *Individual freedom* – means that mentees have some freedom in deciding the amount and type of learning, and patients or service users have a say in the clinical interventions available, where possible.

Other principles of ethics include: (a) autonomy; (b) beneficence (doing good); and (c) non-maleficence (doing no harm). Furthermore, the British Association for Counselling and Psychotherapy's (2010) 'ethical framework' for counselling encompasses values, principles and personal moral qualities. Values refer to respecting human rights and dignity, alleviating personal distress and suffering, and fairness. Personal moral qualities include empathy, sincerity, humility and competence.

Gallagher and Wainwright (2005), reporting on deliberations at the annual RCN Congress, however, indicate that much of nursing ethics are theoretical level academic discourses and do not translate into day-to-day practice and eventualities regularly encountered by healthcare professionals. They suggest that ethics is subjective, and competent ethical practice depends to a good extent on the integrity, honesty and moral behaviour of the healthcare professional.

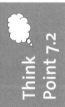

**Think Point 7.2**

## Application of principles of ethics

Think of healthcare professionals whom you know personally, and consider in some detail how far you agree with Gallagher and Wainwright's (2005) suggestions that ethics is much talk and less application. Consider this also in the context of Thiroux and Krasemann's (2007) principles of ethics.

The codes of practice of healthcare professional regulatory bodies often incorporate ethical principles that registrants have to follow. As for mentors' relevant ethical practice in the assessment of competence, they should, for instance, not award a pass to a student for any particular competency if they are not completely sure that the latter can perform the clinical intervention competently.

The NMC (2008a) standards for mentors emphasise effective mentoring practices through the competences and outcomes for mentoring it has identified. For instance, under the domain 'Assessment and accountability', it specifies that the mentor must be competent to 'manage failing students so that they may enhance their performance and capabilities for safe and effective practice' (2008: 52–3). This competence implicitly suggests that mentoring practices must also comply with ethical and legal aspects of both patient or service user safety and care, and of facilitation of learning and assessment of learners' competence.

Furthermore, Duffin (2005) notes that mentors could face misconduct proceedings if they pass students who are incompetent, and that the NMC indicates that they will try to support mentors who feel unsupported if they wanted to fail students. This is because it seems that in the past some mentors felt that they would not be given this support. Giving mentors 'protected time' for mentoring is also again advocated.

One of the legal implications of assessments is that on being awarded a pass, the individual is being given a licence and the legal right to practise the skill unsupervised when they register with their professional body. Awarding a licence to practise to someone who is not competent is technically in breach of the law. The clauses of the NMC (2008b) code of conduct clearly indicate that all registrants (i.e. including healthcare mentors) are personally accountable and answerable for their practice and must 'adhere to the laws of the country'.

A feature that frequently surfaces when the legality of the actions of registrants is questioned is the documentation of the actions taken. The NMC (2009c) and various other authorities clearly believe that if an action is not documented then it cannot be seen as having been performed. For instance, Kendall-Raynor (2007) reports on the case of a registered nurse who had allegedly failed to supervise a mentee adequately, which resulted in the wrong dose of medication being given to a patient, who subsequently died. The case was dropped by the Crown Prosecution Service 'because of insufficient evidence', although it was due to be heard subsequently by the NMC's conduct and competence committee. This is an example of when legal and ethical aspects of mentoring may reflect different perspectives.

All four professional bodies directly involved in health and social care, namely the HPC, NMC, GMC and General Social Care Council, either explicitly or implicitly incorporate such ethical components as respect of patient or service user as individuals, obtaining consent prior to clinical interventions, protecting confidential information, and identifying and minimising risk to patients or service users through their codes of practice.

The principles of ethics translate into current healthcare practice by addressing accountability, informed consent, confidentiality (including record keeping), professional misconduct, delegation and supervision.

## Responsibility and accountability of the mentor

All healthcare professionals are accountable for delivering care competently (NMC, 2008b), and also for other components of their roles such as enabling healthcare learners and colleagues to develop their clinical skills. We are accountable to our patients, ourselves, our employers, our professional regulatory bodies, and in fact also to the general public.

To be responsible implies being answerable for one's actions, and it is a component of accountability. However, Stuart (2007) notes that before the registrant can be accountable, certain preconditions have to prevail, namely: (a) the ability (knowledge, skills and attitude) to decide and act on a specific issue; (b) responsibility; and (c) authority.

One of the main thrusts of the mentor's accountability is that it is related to the rules, regulations, policies and scope of practice that govern assessments. These are usually detailed in the appropriate mentor's handbook issued by the associated HEI, and briefly in the student's practice competencies or outcomes booklet for the placement. It is also related to specific eventualities in the assessment of professional competence, to implementation of assessment strategies, to personal and professional responsibilities, and to the relevant legislation. You would need to refer to the mentee's placement competencies booklet and to your professional regulatory body's code of practice for further clarification when needed.

The healthcare professional's mentoring responsibilities direct the spotlight on one specific area of their several professional roles, that of developing and improving the professional expertise of their mentees.

---

### Activity 7.6   Teaching and learning as components of professional conduct

Refer to your professional regulatory body's code of practice and the partner HEI's mentor handbooks for your own profession, and ascertain how they express your responsibilities in terms of teaching (and assessing) others.

---

You will have noticed that a few clauses in the codes of practice directly identify registrants' teaching and own CPD responsibilities and roles. This is usually also a component of healthcare professionals' job description (or contract of employment) for the post they occupy.

Registrants may not transfer or delegate their accountability to another person. The mentor also functions under legal obligations for knowing about the mentee's course curriculum and built-in assessment procedures and regulations set out by the relevant HEI, and the appeals system that the mentee needs to follow if they feel that they are being unjustly treated. Students have a right to appeal against the conduct of the assessment, but not against the mentor's decision to pass or fail, or their professional judgement about safe practice.

In accepting the role of mentor, the registrant is implicitly accepting responsibility and accountability for maintaining standards of supervision and assessment. The mentor's accountability for student learning is not fully clear, and instances of concern are investigated in their own right. However, the mentor must ensure that students gain the necessary clinical experiences to develop their professional competence and that the mentee does 'no harm' to the patient or service user, by teaching them the correct way of performing clinical procedures.

Rowntree (1987) indicates that there are times when the mentor might intentionally give permission to the learner to perform clinical interventions while supervising them unobtrusively, which can be expected, but at the same time assessing their performance without having specified this to them beforehand. This is sometimes referred to as 'hidden assessment', and could be another instance of unethical action by the mentor.

Furthermore, both initial preparation and continuing development are the joint responsibility of healthcare trusts and HEIs. Making professional judgements about the performance of students, and their ability to provide professionally competent and safe care, constitutes an endeavour to achieve predictive validity and reliability in assessments of competence.

The NMC (2008b) affirms that the interests of the patient or service user are paramount, that is, accountability to the patient or service user is more important than accountability to the student. However, the legal perspective can be, depending on individual situations, that the student is also answerable for incompetent interventions. Lack of experience or knowledge is not an acceptable reason for incompetent care.

On not being awarded a pass for a skill that was not performed competently, the learner might feel either merely disappointed or emotionally distraught. The mentor then needs to contact the PEF or link tutor if further help and support is needed, but might also have to use basic counselling skills (Quinn and Hughes, 2007) to help the learner. As for all professional skills, if the mentor does not feel able to perform these skills competently, then they should refer the learner to an appropriate professional who does have those skills.

## Supporting the Underachieving Student

The mentor's leadership includes careful planning of practice placement to ensure practice objectives are achieved. However, it is well appreciated that, for a number of reasons, some students could be seen as struggling or even failing to show consistent learning and progress during the placement. So what are the different reasons for a student failing to achieve as expected?

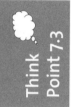

**Think Point 7.3**

## The underachieving student

From your own experience of students who struggle to achieve their clinical competencies, think of the different reasons for this happening during practice placements.

Some students genuinely experience obstacles that intervene in their achievement of placement objectives. Could this be because they are working extra shifts to supplement their income, and therefore are not able to find sufficient time to work on their practice objectives? There can be work-based reasons, or other personal or domestic reasons. The RCN (2007) suggests a number of actions that the mentor should take if his or her student is not achieving the set objectives by expected dates, including meeting with the student as soon as possible to discuss this issue; informing the associate mentor and the designated PEF; constituting a realistic action plan; making provision for any extra support; clarifying the area of weakness and advising on how to progress; and keeping careful notes of all discussions and incidents.

The signs that suggest that a student might not progress as expected with the placement objectives can appear very early during the placement. Limited interaction with clinical staff, lateness, sickness, absent-mindedness, inconsistency in standards of care delivery are just a few of them, but when such signs are detected, prompt actions should be taken.

### Activity 7.7    Failing to fail students

So, for one reason or another, a student might not be progressing as expected, and the mentor is not convinced that particular competencies will be achieved. However, on occasion mentors still decide to pass the student, as found by Duffy (2003).

Consider the whole spectrum of reasons why you think a mentor might award a pass to a student for a particular competency, even if the student has not demonstrated competent performance. List as many reasons as you can think of.

You should have been able to think of various day-to-day circumstances that might lead to the mentor awarding a pass to a failing student, none of which is likely to be a justifiable reason. These could include, for instance, pressure from the student, who indicates that it is the last week of placement and that they have passed all previous placement competencies so far, and insufficient time allocated for assessing competencies.

As indicated earlier, 'failure to fail' has been identified as a dilemma over a number of years (e.g. Lankshear, 1990; Gainsbury, 2010), and can occur in other health and social care professions (e.g. Sharp, 2000). At times, the mentor may have done all the planning for the student to achieve competencies, and yet on assessment they might find that the student has not reached the level of competence required to award them a pass for particular competencies. This could mean failing the practice placement. Consequently, the student's placement may have to be extended to allow them more time to achieve the competencies, and their course extended. Individual HEIs usually provide their own specific guidelines on the actions to take to support the struggling student. The necessary steps in such guidelines are sketched out as a simple algorithm in Figure 7.1.

Although as a compact whole-story process Figure 7.1 constitutes the actions that mentors should take to facilitate learning and achievement for the under-achieving student, each step or stage comprises a concerted intervention that needs to be handled carefully and professionally. Furthermore, some students are likely to become upset or ashamed at failing the placement, or maybe they did all they could but still did not achieve. The mentor will then need to draw on their helping skills to help the student further.

## Helping and counselling the struggling student

The general and specific communication skills needed to establish a relationship and support the mentee develop and achieve competencies were explored to some extent in Chapter 1. In particular, the 'Communication continuum – related skills, and who uses them' detailed by Scammell (1990) (see Table 1.1) suggests that specific communication skills are needed for helping students who are struggling to achieve their clinical competencies, or who may be struggling with the nursing course as a whole and are even in danger of failing in their chosen career.

It is suggested at this point that you refresh your understanding of the communication skills discussed in Chapter 1. In addition to the generic communication skills that are necessary for all effective relationships, specialist communication skills are also required by the mentor to deal with more problematic situations.

| | | |
|---|---|---|
| Student had been welcomed by the team/mentor at the beginning of the placement   → | No →  | Introduce student to all key members of the health and social care team, or give student names of those who he/she should contact to explore their roles |
| ↓ | | |
| Yes | | |
| Initial interview conducted by named mentor, and learning needs and requirements identified   → | No →  | Conduct initial interview the same day and identify learning requirements |
| ↓ | | |
| Yes | | |
| Continuous supervision of skill acquisition, and formative assessment conducted as appropriate   → | No →  | Student should not be allowed to perform clinical interventions completely unsupervised |
| ↓ | | |
| Yes | | |
| Discuss immediately any area of skill acquisition causing concern   → | Not discussed →  | Consult members of the team, or ask line manager/PEF to do so |
| ↓ | | |
| Yes | | |
| If concern persists, formally explore student's perspectives, and consider or revisit learning contract   → | Not done →  | Student could have grounds for appeal against your summative decision. Draw on mentor support, e.g. personal tutor, PEF |
| ↓ | | |
| Yes | | |
| Alert link tutor/team members and PEF of areas of concern   → | No →  | Do so, to provide wider support to student |
| ↓ | | |
| Yes | | |
| Conduct mid-placement interview, including formative assessment as appropriate; document accordingly   → | No →  | Not documented is seen as not done |
| ↓ | | |
| Yes | | |
| If student fails, or is not achieving goals set in learning contract, then compose a targeted detailed action plan   → | No →  | Action plan required for student so that everyone is clear about their responsibilities |
| ↓ | | |
| Yes | | |

*(Continued)*

*(Continued)*

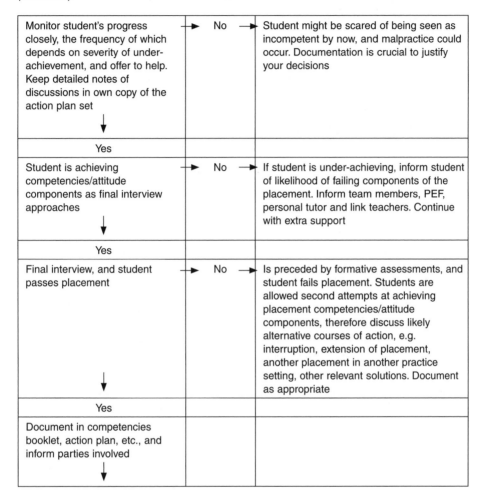

| | | |
|---|---|---|
| Monitor student's progress closely, the frequency of which depends on severity of under-achievement, and offer to help. Keep detailed notes of discussions in own copy of the action plan set | No | Student might be scared of being seen as incompetent by now, and malpractice could occur. Documentation is crucial to justify your decisions |
| Yes | | |
| Student is achieving competencies/attitude components as final interview approaches | No | If student is under-achieving, inform student of likelihood of failing components of the placement. Inform team members, PEF, personal tutor and link teachers. Continue with extra support |
| Yes | | |
| Final interview, and student passes placement | No | Is preceded by formative assessments, and student fails placement. Students are allowed second attempts at achieving placement competencies/attitude components, therefore discuss likely alternative courses of action, e.g. interruption, extension of placement, another placement in another practice setting, other relevant solutions. Document as appropriate |
| Yes | | |
| Document in competencies booklet, action plan, etc., and inform parties involved | | |

**FIGURE 7.1** The underachieving student – actions that the mentor should take

The special skill of 'counselling' is one of the roles of the teacher (Quinn and Hughes, 2007), and increasingly that of the mentor for the reasons just discussed. First, however, it is well recognised that for counselling to be effective the process should be entered into voluntarily by the person being counselled (the counsellee). Indeed, it is generally agreed that unless counselling is actively sought by the counsellee, the interaction might not be as effective, even if the helper uses most of the skills used in counselling. Second, counselling is a therapeutic technique requiring specialist training. Persons not skilled in its use will, at best, not help the counsellee, and at worst potentially compound the counsellee's problems. Therefore, unless they are fully qualified as counsellors, mentors and other teachers in healthcare are more likely to use helping or 'basic' counselling skills. For more intense mentee problems, referral should be made to specialist services such as the university's counselling service, which is usually a section of student services provision.

> ### 🗁 Case Study – The failing student
>
> Bina is a pre-registration student on an eight-week placement at the end of the first year of her course. Her mentor has varied roles as part of their managerial functions, and has to cover extra shifts on days and nights due to staff sickness. However, Bina's placement has been marked by her frequent absence from the practice setting due to sickness, and occasional tearfulness, claiming to feel depressed. She has been advised to seek help from the trust's Occupational Health Department, and has been made aware that she can access the university's counselling facility if preferred.
>
> Shortly after the placement started, the PEF went on maternity leave, and it took a few weeks to install a replacement for her. The acting PEF contacted Bina's personal tutor to explain Bina's circumstances and was advised that, among other things, a mid-placement interview needed to be conducted to ascertain Bina's progress with practice competencies, and documented accordingly. In particular, if these competencies were not achieved, then Bina would fail the first year and not progress to the field-specific part of the programme. The student is described as lacking in motivation and as 'a real struggle' by the acting PEF.
>
> Due to Bina's continuing absence and health problems, the mid-placement interview only took place quite late in the placement, and an action plan was instituted as various practice competencies had still not been achieved.
>
> Consider what would be the specialist helping or counselling skills that could be utilised in regular mentor–mentee contact if both Bina and her mentor were more available.

The most important factor within a counselling situation is the relationship between the counsellor and the counsellee. This was identified initially by Rogers (1983) and later by Rogers and Freiberg (1994), both identifying three key qualities (also known as 'core conditions' of helping) that are required for effective counselling. These key qualities, as detailed under student-centred teaching in Chapter 3, are genuineness, trust and acceptance, and empathic understanding.

In addition to the generic communication skills, verbal and non-verbal, the key helping skills identified by Quinn and Hughes (2007) include self-awareness, attending, active listening, summarising, reflecting, questioning, and using silence. This set of skills can be used as a framework for checking how thoroughly you feel you dealt with these situations. By analysing your interactions with others you will develop a greater awareness of how far you, as a professional, are able to help others.

Dedicated time is required for a systematic approach to counselling. This is done by utilising a model of helping such as Heron's (1989) six-category intervention analysis. This model indicates six possible interactions between the two parties as detailed next. Alternatively, Berne's 'transactional analysis' approach (Figure 1.2) can be implemented.

In the aforementioned case study, for instance, the mentor can help Bina by utilising components of Heron's framework. Instances of responses by the mentor to the student's account of his or her perception of the situation would therefore be as follows:

- *Prescriptive* – advise Bina to reduce less important life activities to concentrate on working to achieve her placement objectives as a priority.
- *Informative* – give information on professional and personal matters as appropriate (e.g. location of Occupational Health Department).
- *Confrontational* – ask Bina directly what she is doing or how she could behave differently for a more amiable experience.
- *Supportive* – allow Bina time and silence to think over the mentor's questions and suggestions.
- *Cathartic* – allow Bina to verbalise and explain in ample detail why she is struggling in this placement.
- *Catalytic* – the mentor acts as facilitator to enable Bina to meet her learning needs.

## Activity 7.8   An underachieving student you have encountered

Think of a student whom you have known to have failed to achieve required practice objectives resulting in the student being disappointed, upset or distressed. In case you haven't encountered such a student, think of a situation that you might encounter. Describe the situation in up to 75 words. Then, utilising Heron's (1989) six-category intervention analysis framework, identify the specific actions that you could take, using each of the categories to help the student.

Alternatively, consider Mel Alexis's situation cited in Chapter 1, and follow the above instructions.

Hawkins and Shohet (2006) suggest taking an inter-subjective approach that focuses on the relationship between mentor and mentee. This notion largely implies using empathy. Universities usually provide a counselling service for any student who is distressed about any issue that is affecting their progress with their course. To become a skilled counsellor, especially for dealing with particular psychological problems, requires several years of structured educational preparation. However, Hawkins and Shohet also provide a number of pointers on how supervisors can help, such as by developing 'the qualities of a good supervisor' in themselves, which are noted in Box 7.5.

---

### Box 7.5     Qualities of a good supervisor

- Flexibility with use of different concepts and intervention methods
- A multi-perspective view (i.e. being able to see the situation from different angles)
- A working map of the discipline or subject area
- The ability to work transculturally
- The ability to contain or manage anxiety of self and supervisee, or refer to an appropriate agency
- Openness to learning from supervision situations
- Sensitivity to the impact of wider contextual issues on the supervision process
- Awareness of different types of power and how to handle them
- Humour, humility and patience

*Source*: Adapted from Hawkins and Shohet (2006)

---

Proctor's (2001) 'supervision alliance model' is widely accepted as a suitable framework for systematic supervision. As a model of helping that is also acknowledged by Hawkins and Shohet, it comprises three main functions or roles of the helper, namely normative, formative and restorative.

Although the mentor is expected to exercise professional judgement and make pass or fail decisions on particular student performances, there are support networks that they can draw on whenever they are unsure. Informal or formal team mentoring and peer consultation frameworks might already be in place, but, as indicated in this chapter, the mentor's copy of the practice competencies booklet normally contains full details regarding the procedure to follow in these circumstances, such as contacting the PEF.

This chapter has explored ways in which the mentor exercises leadership. However, it is useful to note that the leadership role is not just about taking actions to avert problems. It is also about taking actions to achieve aims and good practice. Sines et al. (2006) report on joint actions taken by an NHS trust and the partner university to ensure that student nurses achieve fitness for practice by the end of the three-year pre-registration course. Most of the mechanisms instituted are not unknown, but several of them were planned in substantial detail. These mechanisms include:

- Identifying core skill clusters.
- Adapted OSCEs.
- Enhanced clinical skills laboratories.
- An additional training programme in assessment of skills for existing mentors.
- Regular mentoring updates.
- Appointment of PEF.

# Chapter Summary

This chapter has focused on the mentor's leadership and the challenges of mentoring, particularly in relation to assessments, and has therefore explored:

- The mentor's leadership in careful forward planning of assessments, making decisions and giving feedback to the student after assessing them perform clinical skills. Good practice guidelines for assessments.
- Current criticisms, difficulties and potential problems of assessment of learners' clinical skills, resolving these problems, including action planning and re-assessment of the learner, and how these problems are averted.
- The responsibility and accountability of the mentor in ensuring that a pass or fail is awarded as appropriate, and relevant subsequent actions taken.
- Use of professional judgement, and how intra- and inter-mentor reliability can be monitored and achieved; and the ethical and legal aspects of mentoring.
- How under-achieving or struggling students can be supported using basic communication and helping skills, and more specialist communication skills, including counselling. They constitute skills that would also apply to student assessment situations, and include time management and proactive actions, and the use of support networks with peers, PEFs and academic staff.

# Further Optional Reading

For the full Duffy (2003) and the Gainsbury (2010) reports on failure to fail, see:

- Duffy, K. (2003) *Failing Students: A Qualitative Study of Factors that Influence the Decisions Regarding Assessment of Students' Competence in Practice*. Available at: www.nmc-uk.org/Documents/Archived%20Publications/1Research%20papers/Kathleen_Duffy_Failing_Students2003.pdf. Accessed 23 August 2010.

- Gainsbury, S. (2010) 'Mentors passing students despite doubts over ability …', *Nursing Times*, 106 (16): 1–3.

For principles of giving effective feedback, which is laid out in two columns as actions and rationales, in the format that clinical guidelines are presented, see:

- Gopee, N. (2010) *Practice Teaching in Healthcare*. London: Sage Publications. Table 5.7 'Good practice guidelines for giving effective feedback'.

For more on how to manage failing students in health and social care, see also:

- Marsh, S., Cooper, K., Jordan, G., Merrett, S., Scammell, J. and Clark, V. (2008) *Assessment of Students in Health and Social Care: Managing Failing Students in Practice* (Making Practice Based Learning Work project). Available at: www.practicebasedlearning.org/resources/materials/docs/Failing%20Students-%20final%20version%2022%20Nov.pdf. Accessed 10 September 2010.

The NMC identifies leadership as a domain of activities and specific outcomes for mentors, practice teachers and teachers in supporting learning. Coleman and Glover present an account of what leadership in education signifies, and Chapter 7 presents a useful account of teamworking in education.

- Coleman, M. and Glover, D. (2010) *Educational Leadership and Management*. Maidenhead: Open University Press.

Ongoing international research-based account of leadership traits, theories, etc. is presented in:

- Kouzes, M. and Posner, B.Z. (2007) *The Leadership Challenge* (4th edn). New York: Jossey-Bass.

For an account and analysis of leadership in healthcare, see Chapter 3 of:

- Gopee, N. and Galloway, J. (2009) *Leadership and Management in Healthcare*. London: SAGE Publications.

# 8
# Evaluating Mentoring

## Introduction

This chapter focuses on the evaluation role of the mentor, primarily because not only is evaluation of learning one of the eight domains of mentoring activities identified by the NMC (2008a) – the other seven domains having already been analysed in preceding chapters – but also because it can be a satisfying experience to receive positive feedback on your teaching, and to identify components for further learning. Additionally, taken from the wider perspective of evaluation of mentoring, evaluating covers mentors self-monitoring the effectiveness and quality of all their mentoring activities, and includes monitoring intra- and inter-mentor reliability in assessments, which was discussed in Chapter 7 as one of the likely challenges of mentoring. Evaluation information forms the basis for progressive learning, and therefore also the mentor's own continuing professional development.

The chapter examines reasons for evaluating mentoring activities, particularly facilitation of learning and assessment of competencies, the exact nature of evaluations, frameworks for evaluation and the opportunities that the outcomes of evaluations present.

## Chapter outcomes

On completion of the chapter, you should be able to:

1 Identify and elaborate on a number of reasons for evaluating such mentoring activities as facilitation of learning and assessment of competence.
2 Explain the nature and various features of evaluation, and who are involved in evaluating mentoring activities.
3 Identify different ways of evaluating clinically based and academically based teaching and assessment.

4  Justify the actions that should be taken following evaluations and the likely difficulties and opportunities presented by them.
5  Explain how the challenges encountered by mentors also comprise opportunities for professional development, as well as for meeting the requirement for continuing learning and updating.

## Why Evaluate Mentoring Activities?

The reason for evaluating mentoring activities is that it is logical to do so to confirm that mentoring practices are, and remain, effective, and to identify likely areas for improvement. As registrants we engage in evaluation of care and treatment continually during any span of duty, and therefore it is not an unfamiliar activity to us. The specific competence and outcomes under the domain 'Evaluation of learning' set by the NMC (2008a) for mentors are as follows:

- *Competence for 'evaluation of learning' domain* – determine strategies for evaluating learning in practice and academic settings to ensure that the NMC's standards of proficiency for registration or recording a qualification at a level above initial registration have been met.

  1  *Outcomes* – (a) contribute to evaluation of student learning and assessment experiences, proposing aspects for change resulting from such evaluation; and (b) participate in self- and peer evaluation to facilitate personal development and contribute to the development of others.

An exploration of evaluation therefore comprises:

- Precisely why we evaluate, what is evaluation, and what does the mentor evaluate?
- Who should be involved?
- How to evaluate?
- What to do with the evaluation data?

---

### Activity 8.1   Why evaluate?

Consider the question why we should evaluate what we do in the course of our duty anyway, and what we can do with information gathered from evaluations. Make notes of your thoughts on this.

---

As noted above, evaluation is an activity that we engage in quite frequently, formally and informally, and at times without realising that we are doing so.

Thus, as with the problem–solving approach in nursing and midwifery, we engage in assessment of patient or service user health problems, plan care and interventions, implement them and later evaluate their effect. Systematic approaches to most novel ventures entail evaluation of the plans implemented, and deciding on the actions to be taken subsequent to evaluation.

There are a number of reasons for evaluation. If mentors do not evaluate their mentoring activities, then they are taking for granted that their actions meet their learners' learning needs. They are assuming that learners are satisfied with the learning provided, and that they are fulfilling their roles effectively. Formal evaluations often reveal unexpected impressions, and therefore the reality might be different. Furthermore, if the mentor or teacher does not evaluate their teaching, then what evidence will they have of their effectiveness? Hence, the NMC's (2008a) requirement for 'Evaluation of learning' is a necessary area of activity for the mentor.

Further reasons for evaluating mentoring activities are:

- To identify improvement points for subsequent mentoring activities.
- To anticipate likely problem areas, and take preventive actions.
- To gauge whether the mentee's learning is pitched at the appropriate level and in appropriate detail.
- Continuing self-monitoring of competence in professional practice is often a requirement of employment.
- It is a component of the practice setting's quality assurance mechanism.
- To gauge progress made.
- It is professional 'good practice'.

In addition to evaluation being performed for the purposes of quality assurance through looking at structures (e.g. resources), processes, procedures, standards and consistency, it is also performed for quality enhancement, that is for improvement through change and development. Evaluation can reveal any problematic aspect and which ones concerned the individual or group of students most, and it can identify areas of confusion or misunderstanding. Consequently, when problematic areas are uncovered, they also present opportunities for creativity, and for novel structures and activities to be suggested and instituted.

Chelimsky and Shadish (1997) identify three levels or approaches to evaluation in that it is performed for: (i) accountability; (ii) knowledge; and (iii) development:

(i) Evaluation for accountability – i.e. to ensure that duties have been performed as required.
(ii) Evaluation for knowledge – i.e. to act on suggestions for extra components or experience to be included in the activity.
(iii) Evaluation for development – actions taken based on evaluation results can constitute growth and improvement for mentor, team members and the organisation.

A fourth purpose can be added in specifying that evaluation is also conducted for management and further development of education programmes. That is, course or module leaders evaluate to identify problems being encountered or foreseen by the students on the education programme, and solving those problems, or averting them. At times, what is seen as an issue just needs further explanation or justifying.

Before evaluation of any activity, it is important to ascertain what the purposes of the activity are in the first place. That is if we are evaluating our teaching, what were the aims of the teaching? The purpose of the teaching will have been to arm the recipient with relevant knowledge and to develop competence, and the purpose of the evaluation would be to check if this has happened. Considering the above-mentioned three approaches to evaluation, is your evaluation of your teaching for the purposes of accountability, to receive suggestions and explore associated ideas, or for management and development of your mentoring activities?

---

### Activity 8.2    Can evaluation of teaching improve learning?

Focusing on the mentor's teaching role, consider the evaluation of teaching that you have experienced, and identify at least two ways in which this can lead to improvement in learning.

---

Healthcare course lecturers are required to evaluate their teaching and act on the evaluation data. Furthermore, as for the evaluation tool used, the NMC recognises that such tools need to be 'fit for purpose', rather than just convenient tools that might be valid ones. 'Fit for purpose' means exactly what the term states, that is, the mechanism has to be appropriate for achieving the objectives of the practice setting or the organisation, and should meet the criteria of the quality assurance framework utilised. Then what do we do with the information about whether or not the knowledge and competence have been acquired?

Following evaluation of teaching, the mentor can follow the teaching component up by offering further reading materials or information to help students meet their learning needs. They can arrange further teaching sessions on topics suggested in the evaluation information, and can also adjust their subsequent teaching with a view to connect more fully with the learner's learning needs.

## What is Evaluation?

Most healthcare professionals are familiar with the concept of evaluation of care, as it constitutes a key component of a systematic approach to care and treatment, and is also an inherent facet of care pathways.

---

### Activity 8.3　What does the term 'evaluation' itself mean?

Make brief notes on what you understand by the word 'evaluation'. What is it about?

---

Evaluation of the effectiveness of care given is important as the goal is to restore health, and we need to know if this has been achieved. Evaluation is also an essential facet of professional education programmes in healthcare in order to review or ascertain how effectively and efficiently the curriculum meets the stated philosophy, aims and objectives of the course. It is a part of the process that reviews the currency and value of the course or module.

The term *evaluation* originates from the French word *evaluer*, meaning to work out the numerical value of something. In current usage in English it means appraising or making a judgement about the worth of something (Brown, 2002: 871). Various definitions of evaluation have been offered by interested parties over the years. For instance, Roberts et al. (2001) indicate that evaluation is essentially about making judgements about the value and worth of something against explicit, justifiable and appropriate criteria. Thus, evaluation is the process of systematically collecting and analysing information in order to form value judgements based on firm evidence.

---

### What do we evaluate?

When evaluating care in clinical practice, exactly what is it that we evaluate, and what are the different ways in which evaluation information is obtained?

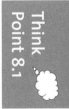

Think Point 8.1

---

Other terms that tend to have similar or overlapping meanings with evaluation are assessment, quality appraisal and monitoring. However, assessment has a distinct and specific meaning in healthcare, referring to assessment of patients' health problems, and of learners' competence. Thus, assessment refers to the collection of data against set criteria. It is therefore objective. Evaluation, on the other hand, refers to the values and personal judgement on whether actions taken enabled the achievement of specified goals.

However, evaluation is also used as an empirical tool in the form of a research method involving in–depth exploration of the component being evaluated through data collection and analysis. In Guba and Lincoln's (1989) fourth–generation evaluation as a research method, the first-generation evaluation is measurement orientated, the second generation is based on measurable objectives, the third generation is judgement orientated, and the fourth generation is based on negotiation. These concepts can be seen as models of evaluation. Redfern (1998) refers to other models of evaluation such as pragmatic evaluation (which begins by ascertaining the practical value of the component), pluralist evaluation (combining several models to form a new one), and realistic model of evaluation (exploring the mechanics of explanation). These concepts may sound a little esoteric to the mentor, but then they do belong to arenas of highly skilled and stringent empirical activities.

Returning to evaluation of mentoring, this can also be public or private, external or internal, continuous or episodic/intermittent and final (refers to time scale). Moreover, evaluation can be case-specific or generalised/holistic, or analytical (see Box 8.1 for a brief explanation of these modes and types of evaluation).

---

### Box 8.1   Who evaluates what?

| | |
|---|---|
| Public evaluation | Open evaluation of an activity by others |
| Private evaluation | Self-evaluation by the person who performed the teaching, for instance |
| External evaluation | Evaluation by others outside the organisation |
| Internal evaluation | Evaluation by departments or individuals inside the organisation |
| Continuous evaluation | Ongoing evaluation |
| Episodic/intermittent evaluation | Evaluation at set or specific times |
| Final evaluation | Evaluation at the end of one or a series of activities |

*(Continued)*

| | |
|---|---|
| *(Continued)* | |
| Case-specific evaluation | In-depth evaluation of one particular instance of an activity |
| Generalised or holistic evaluation | Inviting and gaining overall impressions |
| Analytical evaluation | Detailed evaluation, may include numerical data |

Furthermore, evaluation can be quantitative or qualitative. Generally, for new topic areas, qualitative evaluation is likely to elicit data that can enable further development of the topic. For more established topic areas, quantitative data are sought to monitor or ascertain the likely ongoing effectiveness of the activity.

The evaluation of patient or service user care and of teaching episodes is undertaken formatively and summatively. Formative evaluation of care is a continuous activity, the frequency of which is adjusted according to the dependency level of the patient/service user, or to the criticality of their condition. With some service users who require longer-term care, or those in the community, evaluation may be recorded at longer intervals at specific set periods. Summative evaluations are conducted at end points, i.e. retrospectively, for example evaluation of a practice placement experience, or a module.

Evaluation is also one of the four stages of the regular development review process of healthcare professionals identified in the *NHS KSF* (DH, 2004a). The first stage is the joint review of the individual's work against the demands of the post. This is in the context of the six core dimensions of healthcare work. The second is the personal development planning stage, the third is the learning and development stage, and the fourth is the evaluation stage. At the evaluation stage, the individual:

- Reflects on the effectiveness of their learning and development of their knowledge and skills.
- Identifies how their learning has improved the application of their learning to their post.
- Feedbacks to the organisation on how the learning and development can be improved.

Furthermore, job evaluation is another related concept that is a feature of banding of healthcare professionals' posts under *Agenda for Change* (DH, 2004d).

In the context of evaluating mentoring, this chapter addresses all the above aspects of evaluation except evaluation as a research method. Having examined why we need to evaluate mentoring activities and exactly what evaluation is, it is also important to consider who evaluates before moving on to how mentors evaluate their mentoring.

## Who evaluates teaching and learning?

As mentioned earlier, evaluation can take different forms (see Box 8.1). Formative evaluation of teaching and learning is conducted through informal and formal mechanisms. It is a micro-level evaluation that the mentor performs informally when teaching clinical interventions, either in the clinical area or in university settings. It is a valuable internal mechanism for monitoring one's own competence through a continuous process of observation and sensory feedback.

There is also the formal evaluation mechanism that requires more concrete evidence to be gathered and reproduced when required. Formal evaluation mechanisms can manifest patterns of good or poor teaching delivery. These formal evaluation exercises take place periodically and allow scrutiny of the quality of theoretical and clinical learning. For instance, during the practice placement, the student also engages in a continuous process of informal evaluation of the extent to which the practice setting is also a learning environment.

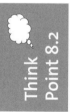

**Think Point 8.2**

## Evaluation of teaching in the practice setting

Who in your experience evaluates the effectiveness of teaching, both planned and informal or opportunistic, in the professional practice setting?

In general, it is the recipient of the teaching, that is, the learner, who is best placed to evaluate the effectiveness of the teaching. Additionally, the result of the teaching will also emerge in the knowledge and skill acquired by the learner and ultimately reflected in the quality of patient or service user care. In addition to the mentor engaging in self-evaluation or self-monitoring the quality of their work-based teaching and assessment, quality and effectiveness can also be ascertained through peer evaluation. Furthermore, evaluation can also be conducted by individual professionals, by clinical teams, or at organisational level.

Generally, there are at least two parties interested in the quality of a service: the provider, and the consumer or user. It seems obvious to suggest that to ensure that consumers get maximum quality from the service, the pro-vider needs to find out first what the consumer wants or needs, and then to be able to deliver the service required. The current purchaser–provider ethos has prevailed in healthcare since the NHS and Community Care Act (DH, 1990). The consumers of mentoring activities are the mentors' learn-ers, and the university whose students they supervise, as well as patients or service users.

---

### Activity 8.4    Who is interested in the evaluation of healthcare courses?

Think of all personnel and agencies that are likely to be interested in the effectiveness and quality of healthcare courses at universities, and jot down specifically who they are.

---

The quality of healthcare courses is of interest to both purchasers and con-sumers of the provision. Purchasers of education are generally students, sev-eral of whom pay their course fees themselves. For healthcare profession courses, the purchaser is the NHS trusts for most pre- and post-registration courses, and individual students based in the NHS or the independent sector (e.g. private hospitals and nursing or residential homes). Other NHS trusts may be regular purchasers of certain courses, as are healthcare students from overseas, and professionals who qualified overseas but are seeking professional registration in the UK. The quality of courses is also of interest to ward man-agers and other qualified colleagues directly dealing with students and who have certain expectations of them during and after the course; and also the public who expects expert professional care.

Strategic Health Authorities (SHAs), and Primary Care and NHS Trusts identify the topic or subject areas of educational programmes required by their healthcare staff to meet the clinical intervention and health needs of the local population. Within a climate of purchasers and providers, educa-tional establishments have to market their educational services and provide evidence of quality assurance measurement within their contracts for serv-ices. Purchasers and consumers can also be seen as users of the service. However, as professional learning takes place in clinical as well as university settings, learning is a partnership agreement between trusts, education pro-viders and students to enable effective delivery of expected professional education.

Other stakeholders interested in the quality of educational provision, as this ultimately impacts on patients or service users' health, are the HEI's internal audit mechanisms, and externally the QAA, the NMC, HPC and other regulatory bodies. Other universities who specialise in education in the subject being evaluated might also be involved. Evaluation by healthcare trusts occurs through feedback from NHS and Primary Care trusts regarding fitness for practice, evaluation of practice placements, and mentors' feedback to the partner university. A number of ways of evaluating education programmes and the various agencies involved in evaluating learning, teaching and assessment are explored in the next section.

## How Mentors Evaluate Learning Provision

Having ascertained why evaluate, what evaluation is and who evaluates, this section explores the different ways in which evaluation is conducted and performed. Broadly speaking, evaluation data can be obtained informally and formally. Informal evaluation can be performed by:

- Direct observation of general state or appearance of a patient or situation
- Direct observation of a class or group of students
- Casual in-class evaluation
- Anecdotal accounts
- Information leaks through the 'grapevine' (the organisation's informal sub-groups)
- Casual quasi-social conversation
- Monitoring whether instructions are being followed

Formal evaluation can be conducted by:

- Assessments, written or oral examinations
- Student surveys – national or local (i.e. at own university)
- Module and course evaluation questionnaires
- Asking the patient directly (or electronically if this facility is available)
- Measurements and pathology laboratory results
- Focus groups

The wide range of learners whose learning the mentor is likely to facilitate includes learners from different healthcare professions and those not following specific programmes of study, and can include patients and their relatives, as identified in Chapter 3. Quantitative and qualitative evaluation information can be obtained through the use of structured or semi-structured forms with selected headings. Such information can also be obtained through verbal or written means. So how do mentors evaluate the more formal practice-based teaching that they deliver?

---

## Activity 8.5    Evaluating facilitation of learning

Think back to a teaching session you delivered recently. You may have taught a student, a colleague or a patient or service user, either a particular clinical skill or a component of knowledge. Which questions did you feel you ought to ask to gain a measure of the effectiveness of the session? Furthermore, exactly how do we evaluate a formal teaching session? What are the methods and set of criteria available to the mentor?

---

Teachers are aware that one of the key elements of any teaching session or learning provision is its evaluation. The teaching session in the practice setting can be evaluated from a number of viewpoints or conducted in various ways. As an internal evaluation mechanism, the teacher (i.e. the mentor) can decide which evaluation tool or model is the most appropriate to gain the necessary information. Some of these tools are identified in Box 8.2.

---

## Box 8.2    Methods of evaluation of teaching in the practice setting

- General discussion at the end of the session
- Verbal feedback – requested/volunteered
- Verbal question and answers
- Feedback from the university, probably through link tutors or PEFs from the particular module leader
- Feedback from colleagues or peers, witness statement
- Quiz – on paper/verbal
- Observing how other teachers teach the skill
- Self-evaluation/reflection
- Using questionnaire(s)
- Observing/monitoring clinical skill performance – direct and indirect
- Continuous monitoring of student's general clinical competence and motivation to learn
- Checking whether objectives are being met
- Reflection/reflective account
- A short multiple-choice-type test
- Discussing booklet of competencies
- Asking the student to teach others, e.g. a patient or junior staff
- Service user feedback
- Using evaluation form(s)

However, evaluation is not always a favoured exercise as, according to Handy (1989), highest-quality service is not easily achieved, since it needs the right equipment, the right people and the right environment, which might not always be fully available. It engenders opinions from all interested parties, who might also set new personal or organisational goals for changing educational provision.

## Evaluating learning using models of evaluation

There are several published or internally designed frameworks for evaluation that individuals or organisations can use for evaluating the quality of learning provision systematically. Maxwell's (1984) six elements or dimensions of quality, is one of them. The six dimensions are: accessibility, acceptability, and appropriateness (3 As), and efficiency, effectiveness and equity (3 Es). Healthcare course providers can develop their own criteria using Maxwell's model for formal evaluation of quality of learning by asking questions related to each of the six dimensions, such as whether the provision was appropriate, efficient, etc. The education provider that aims and claims to offer a quality service should meet all these criteria. Some manage to do so explicitly, while others may be at different stages of development.

Another framework is provided by Lang's (1976) model of quality assurance. This model emphasises the process through a problem-solving approach. Yet another is the popular Donabedian (1988) model of quality assurance using standard statements, and structure, process and outcome components (e.g. Page, 2001). This model was also discussed in the context of practice development in Chapter 5, and the evaluator may choose to evaluate all three components, or only the process component, or outcome.

Mentors, nurse lecturers and other education facilitators can use the Donabedian model to evaluate their learning facilitation. However, university modules and courses are generally evaluated using items under standard headings such as teaching, assessment and feedback, academic support, organisation and management, resources, personal development, and any other comments.

Yet another model of evaluation, which is also utilised as a strategy for management of change, as noted in Chapter 5, involves a cycle consisting of: Plan–Do–Study–Act (PDSA) (IHI, 2010). PDSA comprises a useful framework for evaluation of any new activity in health and social care, and van Epps et al. (2006), for instance, demonstrate the use of a similar framework referred to as 'plan–do–check–act' to evaluate a mentorship programme. The model is usually presented as a cycle made up of four arcs, each beginning with one of the four steps, and thereby meant to represent a 'complete' model. Action research can also be similarly utilised.

## Evaluating professional healthcare courses

Before starting to examine how healthcare courses are scrutinised for whether they meet quality and 'fitness for purpose' standards, it is useful to remember the quality of patients and service user care itself is closely scrutinised regularly by appropriately appointed organisations. Such organisations, which are legally empowered to monitor and periodically measure the quality of service being provided, have their own framework and set of criteria for arriving at a decision as to whether the service meets the government's and the public's expectations.

Currently in the UK, health and social care services are 'inspected' through 'special reviews' by the Care Quality Commission (2010) who judge quality of care utilising 'essential standards' as criteria. The six specific areas of standards that the Commission focuses on are:

- Information and involvement
- Personalised care, treatment and support
- Safeguarding and safety
- Suitability of staffing
- Quality and management
- Suitability of management

There are a number of outcomes under each of these six areas, such as 'meeting nutritional needs' that comes under 'Personalised care, treatment and support'; and 'cleanliness and infection control' under 'Safeguarding and safety'. However, for evaluating educational preparation programme for healthcare professionals, different headings and outcomes are necessary.

---

## Activity 8.6   Evaluating academic programmes

Consider education provision as a public service provided by a particular university with which you are familiar. What criteria would you personally use to judge the quality of their education programmes? Make a list of these criteria. Now try and identify issues or aspects that constitute good quality education provision, say in relation to a course you are interested in, in the health or social care department of the university.

If available, obtain local or national criteria, say from the internet, that could be used to ascertain the quality of this service. Do they match your own criteria of quality, and do any of these standards match the services which are actually being provided?

The QAA (2009) conducts audits of the quality and standard of universities' educational programmes, including those of healthcare education programmes. These audits (or evaluations) are referred to as institutional audits or major reviews, and for these, the QAA utilises its own evaluation framework and criteria. The Department of Health, through a partnership comprising the NMC, the HPC and the SHAs, also carries out reviews of all NHS-funded healthcare education programmes regularly, and has its own framework and criteria for doing so.

The QAA indicates that it's 'mission is to safeguard the public interest in sound standards of higher education (HE) qualifications and to inform and encourage continuous improvement in the management of the quality of HE' (2009:1), which it achieves through institutional audits. The components of the QAA framework are (Section 11):

- *Institutional management of academic standards* – e.g. use of internal and external reviews, and of infrastructures such as assessment policies
- *Institutional management of learning opportunities* – students' involvement in quality management, research activity to inform learning opportunities, learning resources, admissions policies, student support, staff appraisal and support
- *Institutional approach to quality enhancement* – e.g. the academic infrastructure and other reference points, management information, dissemination of good practice, staff development and reward
- *Collaborative arrangements* – e.g. use made of external examiners, and of feedback received
- *Institutional arrangements for postgraduate research students* – e.g. reviews of research provision, of research students
- *Published information* – e.g. accuracy and completeness of published information, students' experience of these related to their programmes of study

The reviewers then deliver one of the following judgements on academic and practitioner standards – 'confidence', 'limited confidence', or 'no confidence'. The above-mentioned audit (or 'subject review') components can be used by universities for internal ongoing evaluation of programme provision in readiness for formal periodic QAA review. The QAA also publishes various guidelines documents which universities can use to gain an impression of the QAA's expectations.

The NMC, on the other hand, performs regular monitoring reviews of nursing and midwifery education programmes through the quality assurance agency Mott MacDonald. In its *Quality Assurance Handbook*, Mott MacDonald (2009) provide full details of the criteria against which they determine the quality of the university's education programmes related to healthcare, which are grouped under the themes:

- Resources – e.g. appropriately qualified nurse lecturers and mentors
- Admissions and progression – e.g. considering health and character of applicants, accreditation of prior learning
- Practice learning – e.g. providing suitable learning opportunities in practice settings
- Fitness for practice – acquisition of required skills and proficiencies
- Quality assurance – programme evaluation, involvement of external examiners, etc.

The quality of the programme is judged on a total of 23 indicators under the above five themes, and the university also has to submit a report for each of its NMC approved programmes to Mott MacDonald every year.

A key component of these reviews (or audits) of university courses is that the reviewers' remits include inspecting practice settings where students gain clinical experience, and this usually includes interviewing mentors and clinical managers. Evaluation requires openness and trust by both parties, a willingness to be open about expectations, and about the strengths and weaknesses in the organisation. Appropriate resources are required to meet the specified standards and consumer expectations and needs.

In addition to Maxwell's, Lang's, Donabedian's, the QAA's and NMC's models or frameworks of evaluation, Dean (2000) refers to the classical evaluation model which specifically includes measurements of the extent to which the learning outcomes were achieved. However, evaluators normally seek quantitative as well as qualitative data by asking for further comments after each question. Furthermore, professional bodies such as the RCN (e.g. *Quality Education for Quality Care: A Position Statement for Nursing Education* (RCN, 2003)), and the Royal College of Midwifery usually also recommend quality improvement measures on specific aspects of practice.

This chapter has so far examined the evaluation of teaching, learning provision and assessment. The next aspect to consider is the destination of the evaluation data.

As for module evaluation, the academic who is the module leader collects information about the module from students against particular criteria such as:

- Staff – whether they were well prepared, accessible, gave constructive feedback
- Teaching and learning methods
- Assessment – marking criteria, feedback
- Resources – teaching rooms, library support, and online support
- The module itself – its relevance, difficulty level, whether the module was well-organised, and achieved its aims and objectives

The module leader has to present evaluation information at academic team meetings, together with the actions being taken to rectify any problem areas identified, and should highlight other key issues. As stated before, the module itself will have undergone quality scrutiny prior to delivery to students. Assessment questions will have been peer reviewed, approved by the relevant internal committee and then by the external examiner. However, flaws in the delivery of the module may surface due to, say, resource problems or with pass rates.

Usually, the module leader also has to report on the number of students who started on the course or module, how many completed on the first attempt, how many dropped out, and how many passed on re-submission. Internal moderators and external examiners report on quality of scripts, and consistency of marking is also considered.

Institutional evaluation issues are actioned or dealt with by heads of department or at Deanery level. Placement issues are jointly resolved by mentors and clinical managers, and university link tutors. Senior clinical managers and higher-level university personnel may be involved in resolving more major issues.

## Evaluating practice placements

Standards of teaching in practice settings are closely related to the quality of patient or service user care, the quality of student supervision, and the expertise of mentors. For students' learning experiences during placements, the student may be asked informally at the end of the placement how good and useful they felt the placement has been, maybe at the same time as the final interview at the end of the placement, or they may be given an evaluation form to complete after the final interview. On returning to the university for lectures after the placement, they are asked to complete a practice placement evaluation form, along with further verbal evaluation.

The written placement evaluation form asks students to give feedback on various aspects of the experience, such as whether they had adequate preparation for the placement, and were given an orientation on the first day of placement. They may be asked to comment on whether a named mentor had been identified, whether their learning needs and placement objectives were agreed in good time, a range of learning opportunities identified, feedback on performance of clinical skills given, how often they worked with their mentor, and whether evidence-based practice was prevalent. There could also be questions on the amount and nature of personal support available.

Evaluation information on the quality of the learning experience is imparted to the placement areas by the university afterwards. The mentor may have obtained qualitative evaluation information from the student prior to the end of the placement. Placement evaluations also form a basis for communication between professionals in practice settings and university lecturers, and an additional benefit of the process is that training and development needs of clinical staff can be identified for both effective clinical care and for competent mentoring practice. Problems reported after the placement are generally investigated by PEFs.

## Evaluation of assessments

The mentor performs numerous assessments of competencies in this role. How are the quality and efficacy of assessments performed by a mentor monitored? The mentor's professional judgement comes into play to some extent, as they have to be able to justify the decisions they make about the student's competence, in that the responsibility normally lies with the mentor to seek all information relevant to assessments, and to keep their own professional competence up to date. Furthermore, if a student feels the result of an assessment was unfair or incorrect, then he/she can appeal following appropriate procedures. This is usually only for the conduct of the assessment and any technical or practical interference during the assessment, but not against the professional judgement of the mentor.

Evaluation of assessment of theory is conducted through structured mechanisms. The pass mark for coursework or assignments for healthcare professional education courses is often 40 per cent. Assignments are marked by module teams, final projects are double marked, and then a stratified sample of scripts is internally moderated by another lecturer in the team, and then further scrutinised by external examiners. All are answerable to assessment or examinations boards and programme boards. Less clear student situations are debated, further advice is sought if necessary, and decisions are made using the university's rules and regulations and professional judgement.

## Evaluating assessments

Consider how the mentor evaluates the soundness of the assessments they perform. How do mentors ascertain that their own knowledge and competence in assessing students remain up to date, valid and reliable?

**Think Point 8.3**

In response to Think Point 8.3 you may have felt that the mentor's accountability has a major role to play in ensuring that their own knowledge and competence in assessing students remain up to date, valid and reliable. This can be achieved by:

- Discussions on mentor update study days regarding, say, intra-mentor and inter-mentor reliability.
- Team mentoring (including assessing).
- Consulting link tutor, PEF and/or senior colleague (e.g. ward sister).

Ways of achieving intra-mentor reliability were examined in Chapter 7.

## Evaluation Results and Development Opportunities

Educational programmes are evaluated by the use of broader generalised forms that can be used for several different courses, by different authorities who use their own set of criteria, as well as by the course or module leader for 'micro-evaluation'. The latter, which Rogers and Horrocks (2010: 284) refer to as case-specific, and analytical evaluation, can reveal honest and more specific individual feelings related to the amount and relevance of teaching and learning, and the learning experience itself. Accurate evaluation is a complex skill to acquire, especially if change is anticipated. It is also often an uncomfortable exercise as it may reveal unanticipated flaws, or perceived flaws depending on the evaluator's own state of mind and general outlook. There might be other biased views stated, or practical problems related to evaluation of teaching highlighted, whether the teaching should be clinically based or classroom based.

Following on from these observations, the next part of this chapter explores problems and the possible consequences of evaluations, and then their likely implications for CPD for mentors. Mentoring RNs on specialist practice courses, lifelong learning, support mechanisms for the mentor, and the use of professional development plans are also discussed.

### Problems and consequences of evaluations

As discussed throughout this book, the mentoring role of health professionals has various facets. Consequently, each facet involves a set of activities in itself, which requires relevant knowledge and competence. To ascertain how well each role is being performed, the mentor has to evaluate and self-monitor their performance, and also obtain feedback from mentees, peers and their own mentors or clinical supervisors. How much and how comprehensively does the mentor do this, and what do they do with the data obtained?

Mostly, this is not an issue because, as an accountable professional, the mentor continually endeavours to rectify any weakness in their performance and knowledge, and strives to enhance their practice at all times. However, there can be problems with the evaluation of mentoring.

## Issues with evaluation

What do you feel are the likely problems associated with evaluation of the mentoring role?

A possible problem area or danger related to the evaluation of a teaching session is that the criticisms of one's earlier teaching sessions may give the impression that you are not quite cut out for teaching. Despite this, teaching is one of the competencies of all qualified nurses and, like many other skills, can be learned and subsequently mastered with ample practice. It is also usually one of the items in the RN's job description, at times worded as 'contribute to professional development of other staff'. On self-evaluation of their mentoring functions (referred to by Rogers and Horrocks (2010) as post-hoc evaluation), they may encounter weaknesses that they may not wish to reveal to others and choose to rectify themselves by trial and error.

Practice placement evaluations could also highlight serious problems with mentoring, as found by Phillips et al. (2000), for instance, that might not prove easy to resolve. The mentor needs to be able to differentiate between progress and levels of attainment by learners. All learners may be making progress but they could be achieving at different levels depending on their educational background, efforts and time for study, and learning opportunities. Some of the likely problems of evaluation are as follows:

- Judgement pronounced can be aimed at influencing peers' opinions.
- Just one incident may colour statements about the whole session, or the module/ placement experience.
- Teacher may be a perfectionist and may feel very disappointed if any weakness is pointed out.
- Points identified by students might not be seen as positive statements.
- May be seen as 'some you win, some you lose', and no action taken on suggested weaknesses.
- The person might genuinely not appreciate the weaknesses pointed out.
- Difficult to be entirely objective.

Research and ensuing recommendations have highlighted problematic areas of mentoring practice and aspects that need developing. For instance, Phillips et al. (2000) identified the role conflict that mentors encounter. Many of the challenges the mentor encounters are related to assessment of practice objectives, and are predominantly due to insufficient time because of having to fulfil their various roles. Many of these issues were identified in particular in Chapter 7 (in Box 7.4).

Furthermore, Gainsbury reports on a problem with assessments that was identified two decades ago by Lankshear (1990), and later by Duffy (2003), but still prevails, which is that some mentors are failing to fail incompetent students. The NMC (2008a) responded to the Duffy report by issuing new standards and other guidelines for mentors; and to the Gainsbury report by reminding universities and their partner healthcare trusts of their account-ability with regards to passing students signifying fitness for practice. Such issues may also present as further professional development requirements for previously qualified mentors.

Duffin (2005) reports that the NMC also remains concerned about the range of clinical expertise in the armoury of the newly qualified nurse, mid-wife or SCPHN, and is therefore considering relaxing the rules on 'skills labs' in which students carry out simulated procedures on dummies. Such labora-tories have almost always been in use but the time spent in them is not gen-erally counted towards the 50 per cent of time that nursing students are expected to spend on practice placements. This issue is addressed by the NMC (2010a) through its declaration that up to 300 of the 2300 hours of practice can be achieved within simulated learning environments, such as in skills laboratories.

The NMC also indicated that: 'We are looking specifically at what might be needed at the point of registration for a nurse in the twenty-first century. Currently, we may well be putting nurses on the register who are not com-petent' (Duffin, 2005: 4). The possibility of incorporating a post-qualifying probationary year for newly qualified registrants is being considered.

In response, university deans of nursing indicated that there was 'evidence that students on placements are under extreme pressure' (Duffin, 2005: 4). The NMC engages with nurse directors and Department of Health officials on how to improve placements, and give mentors 'protected time' for mentor-ing activities. The NMC, however, wouldn't wish to instruct trusts to intro-duce some of these measures, especially when there are major cost implications, but can recommend them.

As just indicated, evaluation of mentoring activities is likely to highlight areas that are problematic or those that warrant further development. The mentor also has a duty to be up to date in all eight domains of the mentoring role. Thus, of necessity, the mentor has to engage in ongoing learning and continuing professional development in relation to mentoring and other roles or dimensions. So, what is continuing professional development (CPD) and what is ongoing or lifelong learning, and how does the mentor participate in these?

## Continuing Professional Development for Mentors

The NMC (2008a) identifies registrants' roles in supporting learning on a continuum that generally progresses as follows:

Nurse or Midwife → Mentor → Practice Teacher → (Qualified) Teacher

Intercalated between these qualification-based positions are likely to be various education facilitation and assessor of competence roles such as sign-off mentor, preceptor, clinical instructor, clinical education co-ordinator and lecturer-practitioner. These various stages constitute the mentor's own ongoing professional development. Therefore this final section of this examination of mentoring and supervision focuses on the scope of the mentor's CPD needs as well as requirements. It suggests in addition to continuing to develop own health or social care practice knowledge and competence, a likely progression for nurses' and midwives' teaching role is to advance from becoming a qualified mentor to sign-off mentor to preceptor to mentoring specialist and supervising advanced practice students to practice teacher and beyond (e.g. nurse lecturer) – as illustrated in Figure 8.1. Annual updates and triennial reviews for mentors (and continuing mentor support – including clinical supervision) as well as being a lifelong learning healthcare professional are the more immediate next steps.

Professional development of mentors as sign-off mentors is dependent upon whether the mentor will be required for supervising final placement students and assessing their 'standards of proficiency'. The signing-off proficiency role of the mentor was examined in some detail in Chapter 6.

The mentor may be required to take on the preceptor role for newly qualified RNs or RNs who are new to the clinical specialism (the preceptor role was discussed in some detail in Chapter 1). They might benefit from availability of clinical supervision. The mentor may also be required to facilitate

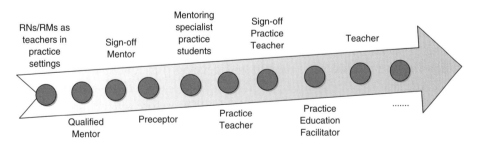

**FIGURE 8.1**  Progressive development of the RN/RM's teaching role

learning and assessing competence for RNs on post-qualifying clinical short courses. Naturally, they will need to hold the same post-qualifying short-course qualification themselves in the first place. However, to facilitate learning and assessing students on specialist or advanced practice educational programmes, they will need to hold the particular specialist or advanced practice qualification, and also have successfully completed an NMC approved, HEI-based practice teacher course.

However, before moving on to these roles, the mentor needs to continue to develop mentoring knowledge and skills, and keep up to date with the latest developments related to the NMC's (2008a) competence and outcomes for mentors. They will have to attend annual updates, and most HEIs, and trusts already have a partnership agreement for such ongoing development of their mentors. This constitutes a programme of learning for qualified mentors, which can incorporate e-learning mechanisms and reflective learning. Mentors who complete these programmes may be eligible for academic credit points. Furthermore, self-evaluation, along with personal research and clinical audits, can highlight issues that can present opportunities for further development for mentors.

As for the mentor's own ongoing professional development, a brief overview of what is continuing professional development and lifelong learning is provided next in this chapter, along with the specific CPD requirements of annual updating and triennial reviews.

## Theories of CPD

Continuing professional development is a concept that is an inherent component of lifelong learning. It can be defined as 'a process of lifelong learning for all individuals and teams which meets the needs of patients and delivers the health outcomes and healthcare priorities of the NHS, and which enables professionals to expand and fulfil their potential' (DH, 1998: 42). At the practical level, Wallace (1999: 28) sees CPD as a 'term given to the learning which takes place in a professional's career after the point of qualification and/or registration'. Wallace prefers to see CPD as identified and intentional learning rather than learning that only comes from the experience of professional practice.

The HPC (2006: 1) defines CPD as 'a range of learning activities through which health professionals maintain and develop throughout their career to make sure that they continue to be able to work safely, effectively and legally within their changing scope of practice'. CPD therefore reflects a responsible and proactive approach to one's own professional learning, and, as McGill and Beatty (1998) note, it involves an attitude to life and work that allows for creativity in one's professional activities.

The means and framework for CPD is also explained by Madden and Mitchell (1993) who suggest that organisations implement one of two main models of CPD: the sanction model or the benefit model. The employing or regulatory organisation that uses the sanction model tends to penalise the individual for not engaging in the necessary CPD. On the other hand, the organisation utilising the benefit model does not threaten with sanctions but reinforces and, where possible, rewards individuals for voluntary or suggested CPD.

Alternatively, Wallace (1999) suggests the statutory, mandatory and permissive types of CPD. Statutory CPD is that which is undertaken as a result of statute or legislation. Mandatory CPD has a similar meaning, in that it is instigated by an official command or instruction by an authority (such as the NMC), and it is therefore compulsory. Wallace identifies the mandatory CPD model as one which suggests that CPD is a mandate by employers or regulatory bodies, which has to be executed but no penalty is attached directly to the individual if not fulfilled. Permissive CPD is one in which the individual has choice.

Most healthcare professions or regulatory bodies have instituted some form of sanction or mandatory model of CPD. The NMC (2008c), for instance, indicates through post-registration education and practice (PREP (CPD)) that every practising nurse, midwife or SCPHN must declare that they have undertaken a minimum of 35 hours of learning activity relevant to their practice during every three-year cycle to be able to renew their registration. The GMC and HPC have similar requirements.

The learning activity for meeting PREP requirements has to be in relevant areas of practice and can be in one or more of the key components of healthcare interventions aptly categorised in the *NHS KSF* (DH, 2004b) as the six core dimensions, namely: (1) communication, (2) personal and people development, (3) health, safety and security, (4) service improvement, (5) quality and (6) equality and diversity, as noted in Chapter 5, and apply to all NHS employees (except doctors, dentists and some board-level managers).

The *NHS KSF* also identifies 24 specific dimensions under *health and wellbeing, estates and facilities, information and knowledge* and *general*, which apply to some but not all jobs in the NHS. More specific details on each of these dimensions of healthcare interventions are presented in the *NHS KSF* document.

However, as the NMC only requires registrants to declare that they have engaged in the required amount of learning activity, PREP in itself does not constitute a guarantee of up-to-date clinical competence. The CPD advocated by the NMC is the minimum requirement for safe and competent practice, but it is recognised that the practitioner generally engages in substantially more learning than this minimum. Relevant university-based courses normally meet the NMC requirement adequately. Furthermore, self-directed or peer-based learning can also easily contribute to these requirements, as identified in the second outcome under the 'Evaluation of learning' NMC domain noted at the beginning of this chapter. Self-directed learning is explained in detail in Chapter 2 under andragogy and the work of Knowles et al. (1998) and Rogers and Horrocks (2010). Peer learning is also well documented, in particular in the context of human and social capital (see, for instance, Gopee, 2002a).

## Annual updates and triennial reviews for mentors

In addition to educational preparation for the mentor role, the NMC (2008a) requires all mentors to attend annual updates to ensure that they remain up to date with contemporary healthcare as well as mentoring practice, and with technical details of the pre-qualifying educational programmes being followed by their mentees, along with their roles and responsibilities within them. The NMC (2009d: 3) indicates that annual update sessions 'must include the opportunity to meet and explore assessment and supervision issues with other mentors/practice teachers (face-to-face) and explore as a group the validity and reliability of judgements made when assessing practice in challenging circumstances'.

---

### Activity 8.7    Mentor's annual updates

- Following completion of a mentor preparation course, you need to be aware of your own CPD in the mentor role. Consider how you can keep yourself up to date with new developments in professional knowledge and competence within your profession in relation to both clinical practice and mentoring. Discuss this with a colleague or your clinical supervisor.
- What would mentors themselves wish to see covered in the annual update study day?
- Think of a number of types of evidence that you as a mentor can provide at the triennial review. Are there any other types of items that other mentor colleagues can provide?

---

Mentor annual update events are usually one-or half-day-long events conducted by PEFs within the healthcare trust premises, or at universities. At the annual update sessions, issues related to reliability and validity of assessments should always be discussed so that a certain level of parity is achieved in the locality, or better still, examined in small group workshops, which could include group activities to explore the exact ways in which intra- and inter-mentor reliability are achieved and monitored. The NMC (2008a) makes some suggestions of activities to include on annual update study days, such as ensuring:

- Knowledge of current NMC approved programmes.
- Discussion on the implications of changes to NMC requirements.
- Opportunity to discuss issues related to mentoring, assessment of competence and fitness for safe and effective practice.

Support mechanisms available for dealing with 'failing students' could be explored, as well as any new NMC rules and guidelines related to supporting learning in practice, and their implications. The NMC (2008a) requires placement providers to hold and maintain a register of current mentors, which is annotated to indicate which mentors are also sign-off mentors and practice teachers. The register also includes evidence of placement areas having sufficient numbers of up-to-date mentors to support learning for students on NMC-approved education programmes.

In addition to annual updating, the NMC (2008a) also requires mentors to be subject to 'triennial reviews'. These include ascertaining during the development and performance review meeting whether the mentor has engaged in mentoring activities, and kept themselves up to date. Mentors should be prepared to provide evidence to their employers and NMC quality assurance agents of how they have maintained and developed their knowledge, skills and competence as a mentor.

Placement providers can therefore consider such evidence of updating as part of the triennial review, for which mentors can compile a portfolio of their mentoring activities, both as a means of effective record keeping and as evidence of meeting the requirements of triennial reviews. Generally, if a mentor has mentored a specified number of students in the preceding three years, regularly participated in annual updates, and is currently on the NMC's professional register, then these could be treated as sufficient evidence for meeting triennial review requirements.

Some healthcare trusts conduct workshops to facilitate building and presentation of portfolio evidence of mentoring activities and updating at triennial review events (e.g. Gover, 2010). In such workshops, attendees can work in groups to identify a range of activities that comprise items that are pertinent evidence of mentoring activities (item 3 of Activity 8.7). In addition to annual updating, evidence could also include annual performance review objectives, achievement of PDPs' objectives, evaluation or feedback from any related presentations (in-house, or at local or national conferences), any EBP initiative implemented or disseminated, etc.

## Mentoring RNs on specialist practice courses

Post-registration students on specialist programmes have particular learning and assessment needs, a dimension which is not usually addressed on standard single-module mentor preparation courses. In the past, before the advent of the current mentoring courses that ensued from the Philips et al. (2000) study, teaching and assessing programmes were twice as long. For specialist community nursing students, assessments were conducted by Practical Work Teachers and Community Practice Teachers (CPT), the educational preparation for which was one academic year long.

After the implementation of the novel mentor preparation course, whether mentors are at degree or Masters level, it was soon realised that it wasn't sufficient to prepare them to assess the specific competencies of students on some specialist community courses (Stevens, 2003; NMC, 2005b). The NMC (2008a) therefore identified the practice teacher role as a role that mentors had to be educationally prepared for supporting practice-based learning for students on these courses, including those on SCPHN programmes. Gopee (2010) translates in detail how practice teachers can fulfil their role effectively, which includes a thorough understanding of all NMC standards and outcomes for practice teacher, and related knowledge base.

Furthermore, the NMC (2007a) recognises that there is likely to be limited opportunity to assess sign-off proficiencies more than once during the practice teacher course, and therefore they recommend a period of preceptee status for newly qualified practice teachers.

## Mentor support with CPD

Usually, all university–healthcare trust partnerships already have an infrastructure of mentor support that has been established. Mentor support implies a network of personnel and other resources that the mentor can access to discuss and sound out the decisions that they are about to make on their mentee's performance of clinical skills, or to consult. Such support is available from peers and colleagues within their practice setting or department, and also from PEFs, link teachers and the student's personal tutor, which invariably result in further learning. Further support can be gained through professional networks, some of which are formed informally at conferences, and when exploring issues at annual update study days.

Clinical supervision is another mechanism that mentors can draw on for regular structured support and for identifying learning. However, one of the key sources of mentor support for CPD is the PEF team, and the study days and workshops that they offer to mentors. Lecturers who teach on the mentor course at the partner university and reflective practice are other mentor support mechanisms.

## The mentor as role model of lifelong learning

To be a role model for mentees, mentors have to be lifelong learners in both professional practice and mentoring. The concept of lifelong learning has been examined with intense attention in some quarters since the 1970s. The Department of Health (1998: 42) sees lifelong learning as 'an investment in quality' and indicates that 'health professionals in all healthcare settings need the support of lifelong learning through continuing professional development programmes'.

---

### Activity 8.8    Why lifelong learning?

List as many reasons as you can think of for healthcare professionals being required to be lifelong learners. How can healthcare professionals achieve lifelong learning? What are the probable problems with lifelong learning?

---

Lifelong learning differs from lifelong education in that while lifelong education refers to learning activities directed by established education institutions, and which normally leads to a qualification, lifelong learning refers to all forms of learning: formal, informal and incidental. Mentors continue to learn and become even more effective as mentors through attending formal annual updating events after successfully completing the initial educational preparation programme to become a mentor; and informally through consulting and advising colleagues such as during peer mentoring; as well as by incidental learning. This means that the healthcare registrant does not only have a responsibility to facilitate the learning of others, but also to continue learning themselves.

The learning activity undertaken is of course also based on self-assessment, and members of healthcare professions need to be responsible for identifying their own learning needs. Indeed, the NMC's (2008b: clauses 3 and 4) code of practice states that 'as a registered nurse, midwife or health visitor, you are personally accountable for your practice and, in the exercise of your professional accountability, must "maintain and improve your professional knowledge and competence"; and "decline any duties and responsibilities unless able to perform them in a safe and skilled manner"'. Thus, healthcare professions explicitly encourage all trained staff to continue the process of

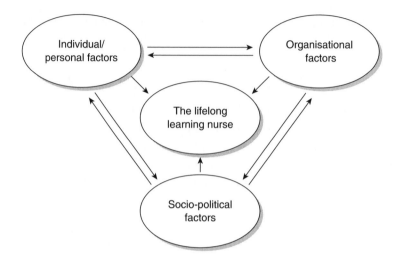

**FIGURE 8.2**   A conceptual framework for lifelong learning in nursing (Gopee, 2005)

learning, asking us to reflect on and question the way we deliver care, and to engage in continuing development of our knowledge and competence.

De la Harpe and Radloff (2000) explored the characteristics of lifelong learning students, and found that these constitute having:

- Self-knowledge, self-confidence and persistence.
- A positive view of the value of learning.
- Good self-management skills, such as being well organised and managing time; knowing when and how to seek help and when to collaborate with peers.
- Motivated to learn.
- Have positive feelings about themselves as learners.
- Able to manage their feelings during highs and lows of learning.
- Have developed a set of learning strategies (e.g. when to dedicate time to study and where to learn; and skills such as note-taking and summarising).

Livneh and Livneh (1999) explored the characteristics of qualified teachers in the USA who regularly participated in learning activities, and found these to be self-motivation to learn, external motivators, as well as situational support and social/environmental resources. As to a systematic approach to facilitating lifelong learning, Gopee (2005) concluded from a qualitative study of nurses' perceptions of lifelong learning that a model (or framework) of lifelong learning in healthcare comprised three groups of factors as presented in Figure 8.2.

In brief detail, these factors comprise:

- *Organisational factors* (e.g. time and release from work to attend CPD courses, work-based learning).

- *Socio-political factors* (e.g. social group influences in the practice setting, clinical supervision).
- *Individual factors* (the healthcare professional's professionalism, learning as a natural human activity).

## Personal development plans

Systematic CPD and lifelong learning for health and social care professionals can also be effectively supported through utilisation of personal development plans (PDPs). PDPs have been advocated for over a decade in the UK through key NHS and education policy documents such as *Making a Difference* (DH, 1999), *NHS KSF* (DH, 2004a), *Guidelines for HE Progress Files* (QAA, 2001) and *The Dearing Report* (NCIHE, 1997). The *NHS KSF* advocates the use of PDPs by all NHS healthcare professionals for their professional development throughout their careers. Other than education and health policies, influential writers on self- and staff management such as Pedler et al. (1997) and Megginson and Clutterbuck (2005) also advocate the use of PDPs.

PDPs provide individuals with the opportunity to focus attention on their career aspirations, and is a mechanism for recording and reviewing career decisions periodically. However, Pedler et al. indicate that PDPs should not be part of the annual development and performance review process which is seen as a management control mechanism, but as agreements that are not centrally recorded. PDPs are instead a component of an effective learning organisation (a concept discussed in Chapter 4).

On the other hand, a PDP is also often an NMC requirement for reinstatement to the professional register where a registrant's competence has been in question, and it suggests that in future, PDPs could be linked to PREP and revalidation. However, a PDP is not a punitive activity, and despite Pedler et al.'s assertion, they can be utilised in conjunction with annual development and performance reviews (Liefer, 2002; Duffin, 2003). It is feasible to implement PDPs so that they are discussed as part of annual development reviews, with only an agreed selection of objectives being incorporated in the performance review, and the remaining PDP objectives being supported by clinical supervision.

The QAA (2001: 8) defines a PDP as 'a structured and supported process undertaken by an individual to reflect upon their own learning, performance and/or achievement and to plan for their personal, educational and career development'. Thus, PDPs can be separated as either personal or professional development, except that for most individuals these two components are either intertwined or experienced on a continuum in day-to-day activities. An example of a PDP for mentors, which has been constructed from prevailing guidance and other literature on the topic, and can be constituted in landscape or portrait format, is presented in Box 8.3.

**Box 8.3  An example of a professional development plan**

Name: ............  [Other relevant details, e.g. clinical supervisor's name]

| Objective and development need/interest | Relevant dimension of my work and career | Hours required and date objective to be achieved | What I will do to achieve this development need/ interest. Resources and support required | How I will apply this learning to my work | How I will know I have completed the development activity successfully | How I will share this learning with relevant others |
|---|---|---|---|---|---|---|
| 1. Establish protected time for mentoring | Teaching learners | One hour every week, achieve by end of mentee's practice placement | Off duty planned in advance. Team members aware. Two alternative protected times identified each week | Spend the protected time to focus on mentoring activities. Monitor and record use of protected time | An appropriate record of mentoring activities | Item on team meeting agenda. Present at local conference |
| 2. Gain practice teacher qualification | ..... | ..... | ..... | ..... | | |
| | | | | | | |

The two development needs mentioned in Box 8.3 are part of the education component of nurses' and midwives' roles, other components being clinical practice, research and management, as noted at the beginning of Chapter 3. Various components of required knowledge and competence can be acquired through in-house and in-service training, but for paid time for study, funding and support from managers for HEI-based courses, this can be an issue (Liefer, 2002), and therefore needs forward planning.

## Chapter Summary

This chapter has focused on evaluation of the whole range of mentoring activities, and having completed this chapter you will have examined:

- Why to evaluate the effectiveness with which mentors facilitate learning and assessments, as well as fulfil other mentoring activities and roles.
- What is evaluation, i.e. the nature and various aspects of evaluation, and who evaluates the mentor's teaching activities?
- Different ways of evaluating clinically based and academically based teaching and assessment; and how mentors evaluate learning provision and assessments during practice placements. The use of models of evaluation, including heeding the findings of audits by external organisations such as the QAA and NMC.
- The likely problems of evaluation, the results of evaluations, issues ensuing from them, related consequences, and subsequent actions that can be taken.
- The opportunities and scope for ongoing learning arising from the results of evaluations, mentoring RNs on specialist practice courses, and the requirement for continuing professional development in one's mentoring role as well as the mentor as a lifelong learner.

## Further Optional Reading

Kirkpatrick and Kirkpatrick's (2005) framework for evaluating training and education programmes is available from internet websites, where they provide variable insights into this model, but a more thorough account is provided in the Kirkpatrick and Kirkpatrick book. Implementation of the model is also discussed in the context of practice teaching in the *Practice Teaching in Healthcare* (Gopee, 2010) book.

- Kirkpatrick, D.L. and Kirkpatrick, J.D. (2005) *Evaluating Training Programs: The Four Levels* (3rd edn). San Francisco, CA: Berrett-Koehler Publishers.

For categorisation of the characteristics of successful lifelong learners in four areas – namely cognitive attributes, metacognitive, motivational and affective – and a discussion on whether and how these characteristics can be assessed, see:

- De la Harpe, B. and Radloff, A. (2000) 'Informed teachers and learners: The importance of assessing the characteristics needed for lifelong learning', *Studies in Continuing Education*, 22 (2): 169–82.

For utilisation/implementation of the Donabedian model of evaluation, see also:

- Page, S. (2001) 'Demystifying practice development', *Nursing Times,* 97 (22): 36–7.

For an identification of sources of mentoring activities that can be presented as evidence/ portfolio evidence at triennial reviews, see:

- Murray, C., Rosen, L. and Staniland, K. (eds) (2010) *The Nurse Mentor and Reviewer Update Book.* Maidenhead: McGraw-Hill Education.

# Further Thoughts – A Journey Just Beginning

Mentoring is a career-long journey, whether it's to do with mentoring learners of one's own healthcare profession, or of allied health professions, medical students, or healthcare assistants. It is a journey that begins soon after your preceptee status ends. One of the strengths of nursing, midwifery and SCPHNs is the holistic approach that other healthcare professionals intend, endeavour and at times succeed in taking in their day-to-day practice. Some clinical settings have students all the time, others occasionally, but the actions that mentors take stay in the minds of healthcare professionals for several years, as they shape their careers and quality of patient care. The mentor's actions are therefore seminal in shaping the attitudes of practitioners for years to come.

On the other hand, as Rogers and Freiberg (1994: 375) indicate, 'not all journeys are trouble-free … but the process alone makes us a bit wiser. Gaining wisdom comes not with time or age, but from living the challenges of life, learning from our mistakes, and building on experiences.' This book on mentoring was designed to achieve the objectives outlined in the introductory section, which is predominantly to examine the knowledge and understanding necessary for effective and mutually beneficial mentoring, and the NMC's (2008a) standards for mentors. The knowledge and skills acquired can be built on by pursuing the topic area further as a part of your own action plan. They could play a significant role along your career path, be it as a more senior clinical practitioner or in part- or full-time educational roles. What are the next steps you'd like to take when you have obtained your mentor qualification?

# References

Anderson, E.E. (2009) 'Learning pathways in contemporary primary care settings – student nurses' views', *Nurse Education Today*, 29 (8): 835–9.

Andrews, M., Brewer, M., Buchan, T., Denne, A., Hammond, J., Hardy, G., Jacobs, L., McKenzie, L. and West, S. (2010) 'Implementation and sustainability of the nursing and midwifery standards for mentoring in the UK', *Nurse Education in Practice*, 10 (5): 251–5.

Anon. (2006) 'Students press for £10,000 a year bursary', *Nursing Standard*, 20 (33): 6.

Argyle, M. (1994) *The Psychology of Interpersonal Behaviour* (5th edn). London: Penguin.

Ausubel, D., Novak, J. and Hanesian, H. (1978) *Educational Psychology: A Cognitive View*. New York: Rinehart & Winston.

Bahn, D. (2001) 'Social learning theory: Its application in the context of nurse education', *Nurse Education Today*, 21 (2): 110–17.

Bailey, M.E. and Tuohy, D. (2009) 'Student nurses' experiences of using a learning contract as a method of assessment', *Nurse Education Today*, 29 (7): 758–62.

Bandura, A. (1986) *Social Foundations of Thought and Action: A Social-cognitive Theory*. Englewood Cliffs, NJ: Prentice-Hall.

Bandura, A. (1997) *Self-Efficacy – The Exercise of Control*. New York: W H Freeman.

Barnett, J.E. (2008) 'Mentoring, boundaries, and multiple relationships: Opportunities and challenges', *Mentoring & Tutoring: Partnership in Learning*, 16 (1): 3–16.

Baron, S. (2009) 'Evaluating the patient journey approach to ensure health care is centred on patients', *Nursing Times*, 105 (22): 20–3.

Barr, H. (2003) 'Interprofessional issues and work based learning', in J. Burton and N. Jackson (eds), *Work Based Learning in Primary Care*. Oxford: Radcliffe Medical.

Barton, T. D. (2006) 'Clinical mentoring of nurse practitioners: The doctors' experience', *British Journal of Nursing*, 15 (15): 820–4.

Bayley, M. and Bayliss-Pratt, L. (2010) Keynote presentation at *Preceptorship: Royal College of Nursing Partners in Practice Conference*. Blackpool, 26–7 February.

Benner, P. (2001) *From Novice to Expert: Excellence and Power in Clinical Nursing Practice*. London: Addison-Wesley.

Berger, P. and Luckmann, T. (1967) *The Social Construction of Reality*. Middlesex: Penguin Books.

Bergsteiner, H., Avery, G.C. and Neumann, R. (2010) 'Kolb's experiential learning model: Critique from a modelling perspective', *Studies in Continuing Education*, 32 (1): 29–46.

Berne, E. (1975) *What Do You Say After You Say Hello?* London: Corgi.

Biggs, J. and Tang, C. (2007) *Teaching for Quality Learning at University* (3rd edn). Maidenhead: Open University Press.

Billay, D.B. and Yonge, O. (2004) 'Contributing to the theory development of preceptorship', *Nurse Education Today*, 24 (7): 566–74.

Binnie, A. and Titchen, A. (1999) *Freedom to Practice: The Development of Patient-centred Nursing*. Edinburgh: Butterworth-Heinemann.

Bloom, B. (1956) *Taxonomy of Educational Objectives: The Classification of Educational Goals, Handbook One: Cognitive Domain*. London: Longman.

Bondy, K.N. (1983) 'Criterion-referenced definitions for rating scales in clinical evaluation', *Journal of Nursing Education*, 22 (9): 376–82.

Boud, D. (1991) *Implementing Student Self-assessment (HERDSA Green Guide No 5)*. Australian Capital Territory, Australia: Higher Education Research and Development Society of Australasia.

Boud, D., Keogh, R. and Walker, D. (eds) (1985) *Reflection: Turning Experience into Learning*. London: Kogan Page.

Bowker, P., French, D., Atkin, S.L., Patmore, J.E., Walton, C. and Aye, M. (2005) 'Financing a diabetes network: Care pathway based costing model for Type 1 diabetes mellitus', *Diabetic Medicine*, 23 (Suppl. 2): 107.

Bradshaw, A. (1997) 'Defining "competency" in nursing (part 1): A policy review', *Journal of Clinical Nursing*, 6 (5): 347–54.

British Association for Counselling and Psychotherapy (2010) *Ethical Framework for Good Practice in Counselling & Psychotherapy* (revised edn). Available at: www.bacp.co.uk/admin/structure/files/pdf/566_ethical%20framework%20feb2010.pdf. Accessed 16 May 2010.

Brooke, J. and Ham, A. (2003) 'Coaching managers to become better team leaders', *Strategic Communication Management (SCM)*, 7 (2): 4–27.

Brown, J., Bullock, D. and Grossberg, S. (1999) 'How the basal ganglia use parallel excitatory and inhibitory learning pathways to selectively respond to unexpected rewarding cues', *Journal of Neuroscience*, 19 (23): 10502–11.

Brown, L. (editor-in-chief) (2002) *Shorter Oxford English Dictionary* (5th edn). Oxford: Oxford University Press.

Brown, L. (2005) 'Ethics in clinical education', in M. Rose and D. Best (eds), *Transforming Practice Through Clinical Education, Professional Supervision and Mentoring*. Edinburgh: Elsevier Churchill Livingstone.

Bruner, J. (1960) *The Process of Education*. Cambridge, MA: Harvard University Press.

Bryar, R.M. and Griffiths, J.M. (eds) (2003) *Practice Development in Community Nursing*. London: Arnold.

Budgen, C. and Gamroth, L. (2008) 'An overview of practice education models', *Nurse Education Today*, 28 (3): 273–83.

Burgoyne, J. and Reynolds, M. (eds) (1997) *Management Learning: Integrating Perspectives in Theory and Practice*. London: Sage.

Burnard, P. and Chapman, C. (1990) *Nurse Education: The Way Forward*. London: Scutari Press.

Care Quality Commission (2010) *Focused on Better Care – Annual Report and Accounts 2009/10*. Available at: www.cqc.org.uk/_db/_documents/CQC_Annual_Report_2009-10_WEB.pdf. Accessed 30 July 2010.

Carlisle, C., Calman, L. and Ibbotson, T. (2009) 'Practice-based learning: The role of practice education facilitators in supporting mentors', *Nurse Education Today*, 29 (7): 715–21.

Carnwell, R., Baker, S., Bellis, M. and Murray, R. (2007) 'Managerial perceptions of mentor, lecturer practitioner and link tutor roles', *Nurse Education Today*, 27 (8): 923–32.

Carper, B. (1978) 'Fundamental patterns of knowing in nursing', *Advances in Nursing Science*, 1 (1): 13–23.

Castledine, G. (1998) *Writing, Documentation and Communication for Nurses*. London: Mark Allen.

Centre for Advancement of Interprofessional Education (CAIPE) (2010) *Defining IPE – Interprofessional Education*. Available at: www.caipe.org.uk/about-us/defining-ipe/. Accessed 29 May 2010.

Chalmers, H., Swallow, V. and Miller, J. (2001) 'Accredited work-based learning: An approach for collaboration between higher education and practice', *Nurse Education Today*, 21 (8): 597–606.

Chartered Society of Physiotherapy (CSP) (2002) *Curriculum Framework for Qualifying Programmes in Physiotherapy*. Available at: www.csp.organisations.uk/uploads/documents/CFforQSP.pdf. Accessed 14 June 2007.

Chartered Society of Physiotherapy (2004) *Accreditation of Clinical Educators Scheme Guidance (ACE)*. Available at: www.csp.org.uk/uploads/documents/csp_ace_scheme_guidance.pdf. Accessed 9 May 2010.

Chartered Society of Physiotherapy (2007) *Accreditation is ACE*. Available at: www.csp.org.uk/director/members/newsandanalysis/frontlinemagazine/archiveissues.cfm?ITEM_ID=CF6BF20FCE8C59A3BDD6A7E3F8D86862&article= (Issue: 18 July 2007). Accessed 31 August 2010.

Chelimsky, E. and Shadish, W. (1997) *Evaluation for the 21st Century – A Handbook*. London: Sage Publications.

Clarke, J.B. (1999) 'Evidence-based practice: A retrograde step? The importance of pluralism in evidence generation for the practice of healthcare', *Journal of Clinical Nursing*, 8 (1): 89–94.

Coleman, M. and Glover, D. (2010) *Educational Leadership and Management*. Maidenhead: Open University Press.

College of Occupational Therapists (COT) (2006) *The Preceptorship Training Manual – A Resource for Occupational Therapists*. London: COT.

College of Occupational Therapists (2009) *Preceptorship Handbook for Occupational Therapists* (2nd edn). London: COT.

College of Operating Department Practitioners (CODP) (2009) *Standards, Recommendations and Guidance for Mentors and Practice Placements. Supporting Pre-Registration Education in Operating Department Practice Provision*. Available at: www.codp.org.uk/Files/CODP%20Standards,%20recommendations%20and%20guidance%20for%20mentors%20and%20practice%20placements_20100101.pdf. Accessed 4 January 2010.

College of Radiographers (2006) *The Approval and Accreditation of Educational Programmes and Professional Practice: Practice Educator Accreditation Scheme*. Available at: www.sor.org/public/practice-educator/pdf/practice-educator.pdf. Accessed 5 June 2010.

Collinson, G. (2000) 'Encouraging the growth of the nurse entrepreneur', *Professional Nurse*, 15 (6): 365–7.

Connor, M. and Pokora, J. (2007) *Coaching and Mentoring at Work: Developing Effective Practice*. Berkshire: Open University Press.

Cross, K.D. (1996) 'An analysis of the concept facilitation', *Nurse Education Today*, 16 (5): 350–5.

Curzon, L.B. (2003) *Teaching in Further Education* (6th edn). London: Continuum.

Dale, A.E. (2006) 'Determining guiding principles for evidence-based practice', *Nursing Standard*, 20 (25): 41–6.

Daloz, L.A. (1989) *Effective Teaching and Mentoring: Realizing the Transformational Power of Adult Learning Experiences*. San Francisco, CA: Jossey-Bass.

Darling, L.A.W. (1984) 'What do nurses want in a mentor?', *Journal of Nursing Administration*, 14 (10): 42–4.

Darling, L.A.W. (1985) 'What to do about toxic mentors?', *Journal of Nursing Administration*, 15 (5): 43–4.

Davies, S. and Priestley, M.J. (2006) 'A reflective evaluation of patient handover practices', *Nursing Standard*, 20 (21): 49–52.

De la Harpe, B. and Radloff, A. (2000) 'Informed teachers and learners: The importance of assessing the characteristics needed for lifelong learning', *Studies in Continuing Education*, 22 (2): 169–82.

Dean, J. (2000) 'The nature and purpose of evaluation', in P. Nicklin and N. Kenworthy (eds), *Teaching and Assessing in Nursing Practice: An Experiential Approach*. London: Baillière Tindall.

Department of Health (DH) (1990) *NHS and Community Care Act*. London: HMSO.

Department of Health (DH) (1996) *Promoting Clinical Effectiveness: A Framework for Action in and through the NHS*. London: HMSO.

Department of Health (DH) (NHS Executive) (1998) *A First Class Service: Quality in the New NHS*. London: DH.

Department of Health (DH) (1999) *Making a Difference: Strengthening the Nursing, Midwifery and Health Visiting Contribution to Health and Health Care*. London: DH.

Department of Health (DH) (and English National Board for Nursing, Midwifery and Health Visiting) (2001a) *Preparation of Mentors and Teachers: A New Framework of Guidance*. Available at: www.dh.gov.uk/en/Publicationsandstatistics/Publications/PublicationsPolicyAndGuidance/DH_4007606. Accessed 11 May 2010.

Department of Health (DH) (and English National Board for Nursing, Midwifery and Health Visiting) (2001b) *Placements in Focus: Guidance for Education in Practice for Health Care Professions*. Available at: www.dh.gov.uk/en/Publicationsandstatistics/Publications/PublicationsPolicyAndGuidance/DH_4009511. Accessed 4 January 2010.

Department of Health (DH) (2001c) *Working Together – Learning Together: A Framework for Lifelong Learning for the NHS*. London: DH.

Department of Health (DH) (2002a) *Liberating the Talents: Helping Primary Care Trusts and Nurses to Deliver the NHS Plan*. Available at: www.dh.gov.uk/cno/liberatingtalents.htm. Accessed 14 June 2007.

Department of Health (DH) (2002b) *PL CNO (2002) 5: Implementing the NHS Plan – Ten Key Roles for Nurses*. Available at: www.dh.gov.uk/PublicationsAndStatistics/ LettersAndCirculars/ProfessionalLetters/ChiefNursingOfficerLetters. Accessed 14 June 2007.

Department of Health (DH) (2004a) *The NHS Knowledge and Skills Framework (NHS KSF) and the Development Review Process*. Available at: www.dh.gov.uk/en/Publications

andstatistics/Publications/PublicationsPolicyAndGuidance/DH_4090843. Accessed 6 April 2009.

Department of Health (DH) (2004b) *Patient Pathways: What Is a Patient Pathway?* Available at: www.dh.gov.uk/PolicyAndGuidance/OrganisationPolicy/Secondary Care/Treatment Centre.html. Accessed 14 June 2007.

Department of Health (DH) (2004c) *European Working Time Directive.* Available at: www.dh.gov.uk/Home/fs/en. Accessed 14 June 2007.

Department of Health (DH) (2004d) *Agenda for Change: What Will It Mean For You? A Guide for Staff.* Available at: www.dh.gov.uk/en/Publicationsandstatistics/Publications/PublicationsPolicyAndGuidance/DH_4090842. Accessed 4 August 2010.

Department of Health (DH) (2006) *Modernising Nursing Careers: Setting the Direction.* Available at: www.dh.gov.uk/en/Publicationsandstatistics/Publications/PublicationsPolicyAndGuidance/DH_4138756. Accessed 8 October 2010.

Department of Health (DH) (2008a) *High Quality Care For All – NHS Next Stage Review Final Report.* Available at: www.dh.gov.uk/en/Publicationsandstatistics/Publications/ PublicationsPolicyAndGuidance/DH_085825. Accessed 8 July 2008.

Department of Health (DH) (2008b) *Common Learning in Health Professional Courses at Coventry University.* Available at: www.hss.coventry.ac.uk/firstwave. Accessed 14 June 2007.

Department of Health (DH) (2008c) *National Service Framework for Long-term Neurological Conditions – National Support for Local Implementation 2008.* Available at: www.dh.gov. uk/prod_consum_dh/groups/dh_digitalassets/@dh/@en/documents/digitalasset/ dh_084580.pdf. Accessed 20 July 2010.

Department of Health (DH) (2009) *Local Routes: Guidance for Developing Alcohol Treatment Pathways.* Available at: www.dh.gov.uk/prod_consum_dh/groups/dh_digitalassets/ documents/digitalasset/dh_110422.pdf. Accessed 2 August 2010.

Department of Health (DH) (2010a) *Preceptorship Framework for Newly Registered Nurses, Midwives and Allied Health Professionals.* Available at: www.dh.gov.uk/prod_consum_ dh/groups/dh_digitalassets/@dh/@en/@abous/documents/digitalasset/dh_114116. pdf. Accessed 24 May 2010.

Department of Health (DH) (2010b) *Equity and Excellence: Liberating the NHS.* Available at: www. dh.gov.uk/en/Publicationsandstatistics/Publications/PublicationsPolicyAndGuidance/ DH_117353. Accessed 24 May 2010.

Department of Health (DH) (2010c) *Health Technology Assessment Programme.* London: DH.

Department of Health (DH) (2010d) *Quality, Innovation, Productivity and Prevention (QIPP) – Case Studies.* Available at: www.dh.gov.uk/en/Healthcare/Qualityandproductivity/ DH_118202. Accessed 31 August 2010.

Dewar, B.J. and Walker, E. (1999) 'Experiential learning: issues for supervision', *Journal of Advanced Nursing,* 30 (6): 1459–67.

Donabedian, A. (1988) 'The quality of care: How can it be assessed?', *American Journal of Public Health,* 260 (12): 1743–48.

Donaldson, I. (1992) 'The use of learning contracts in the clinical area', *Nurse Education Today,* 12 (6): 431–6.

Donaldson, J.H. and Carter, D. (2005) 'The value of role modelling: Perceptions of undergraduate and diploma nursing (adult) students', *Nurse Education in Practice,* 5 (6): 353–9.

Dougherty, L. and Lister, S. (eds) (2008) *The Royal Marsden Hospital Manual of Clinical Nursing Procedures* (8th edn). Oxford: Blackwell.

Duers, L.E. and Brown, N. (2009) 'An exploration of student nurses' experiences of formative assessment', *Nurse Education Today*, 29 (6): 654–9.

Duffin, C. (2003) 'Trusts miss deadline for staff development plans', *Nursing Standard*, 17 (16): 6.

Duffin, C. (2005) 'Pre-registration education to undergo major review', *Nursing Standard*, 19 (26): 4.

Duffy, K. (2003) *Failing Students: A Qualitative Study of Factors that Influence the Decisions Regarding Assessment of Students' Competence in Practice*. Available at: www.nmc-uk.org/Documents/Archived%20Publications/1Research%20papers/Kathleen_Duffy_Failing_Students2003.pdf. Accessed 23 August 2010.

Egan, G. (2002) *The Skilled Helper: A Problem-management and Opportunity-development Approach to Helping*. Pacific Grove, CA: Brooks/Cole.

Entwistle, N. (1994) *Supporting Effective Learning: A Research Perspective*. Edinburgh: University of Edinburgh.

Equality Challenge Unit (2010) *Equality Act 2010: Implications for higher education institutions*. Available at: www.ecu.ac.uk/publications/equality-act-2010. Accessed 23 November 2010.

Evans, D. (2003) 'Hierarchy of evidence: A framework for ranking evidence evaluating healthcare interventions', *Journal of Clinical Nursing*, 12 (1): 77–84.

Falchikov, N. (1986) 'Product comparisons and process benefits of collaborative peer group and self assessment', *Assessment and Evaluation in Higher Education*, 11 (2): 146–66.

Faugier, J. (2005a) 'Reality check', *Nursing Standard*, 19 (19): 14–15.

Faugier, J. (2005b) 'Developing a new generation of nurse entrepreneurs', *Nursing Standard*, 19 (30): 49–53.

Field, J. (1999) 'Participation under the magnifying glass', *Adults Learning*, 11 (3): 10–13.

Fitts, P. M. and Posner, M.I. (1973) *Human Performance*. London: Prentice-Hall.

Flanagan, J., Baldwin, S. and Clarke, D. (2000) 'Work-based learning as a means of developing and assessing nursing competence', *Journal of Clinical Nursing*, 9 (3): 360–8.

Fleming, S., Mckee, G. and Huntley-Moore, S. (2011) 'Undergraduate nursing students' learning styles: A longitudinal study', *Nurse Education Today*, 31, in press, doi:10.1016/j.nedt.2010.08.005.

Freeth, D. and Nicol, M. (1998) 'Learning clinical skills: An interprofessional approach', *Nurse Education Today*, 18 (6): 455–61.

Freire, P. (1996) *Pedagogy of the Oppressed*. London: Penguin.

Fretwell, J.E. (1980) 'An inquiry into the ward learning environment', *Nursing Times*, 76 (16): 69–75.

Fulton, J., Bøhler, A., Hansen, G.S., Kauffeldt, A., Welander, E., Santos, M.R., Reis, M., Thorarinsdottir, K. and Ziarko, E. (2007) 'Mentorship: An international perspective', *Nurse Education Today*, 7 (6): 399–406.

Furlong, J. and Maynard, T. (1995) *Mentoring Student Teachers*. London: Routledge.

Gagné, R. (1983) *The Conditions of Learning and Theory of Instruction* (4th edn). New York: Holt, Rinehart & Winston.

Gainsbury, S. (2010) 'Mentors passing students despite doubts over ability', *Nursing Times*, 106 (16): 1–3.

Gallagher, A. and Wainwright, P. (2005) 'The ethical divide', *Nursing Standard*, 20 (7): 22–5.

Garbett, R. and McCormack, B. (2002) 'A concept analysis of practice development', *NTresearch*, 7 (2): 87–100.

Garside, J., Nhemachena, J.Z., Williams, J. and Topping, A. (2009) 'Repositioning assessment: Giving students the "choice" of assessment methods', *Nurse Education in Practice*, 9 (2): 141–8.

Garvey, B., Stokes, P. and Megginson, D. (2009) *Coaching and Mentoring: Theory and Practice*. London: SAGE.

General Medical Council (GMC) (2010) *Glossary of Terms Used in Fitness to Practise Actions*. Available at: www.gmc-uk.org/Glossary_of_Terms_used_in_Fitness_to_Practise_Actions.dot.pdf_25416199.pdf. Accessed 23 April 2010.

Ghazi, F. and Henshaw, L. (1998) 'How to keep student nurses motivated', *Nursing Standard*, 13 (8): 43–8.

Gibbs, G. (1988) *Improving the Quality of Student Learning*. Bristol: Technical Education Services.

Gilmour, J.A., Kopeiki, A. and Douché, J. (2007) 'Student nurses as peer-mentors: Collegiality in practice', *Nurse Education in Practice*, 7 (1): 36–43.

Goldsmith, J., Clarke, B. and Cross, S. (2009) 'The art of learning to teach interprofessionally', *Practice Nursing*, 20 (8): 414–16.

Gopee, N. (2000) 'Self-assessment and the concept of the lifelong learning nurse', *British Journal of Nursing*, 9 (11): 724–9.

Gopee, N. (2001) 'The role of peer assessment and peer review in nursing', *British Journal of Nursing*, 10 (2): 115–21.

Gopee, N. (2002a) 'Human and social capital as facilitators of lifelong learning in nursing', *Nurse Education Today*, 22 (8): 608–16.

Gopee, N. (2002b) 'Demonstrating critical analysis in academic assignments', *Nursing Standard*, 16 (35): 45–52.

Gopee, N. (2005) 'Facilitating the implementation of lifelong learning in nursing', *British Journal of Nursing*, 14 (14): 761–7.

Gopee, N. (2010) *Practice Teaching in Healthcare*. London: Sage Publications.

Gopee, N. and Galloway, J. (2009) *Leadership and Management in Healthcare*. London: Sage Publications.

Gopee, N., Tyrell, A., Raven, S., Thomas, K. and Hari, T. (2004) 'Effective clinical learning in primary care settings', *Nursing Standard*, 18 (37): 33–7.

Gover, S. (2010) 'Triennial review workshops facilitated by practice education facilitators'. Paper presented at Royal College of Nursing Education Forum *Partners in Practice* Conference, Blackpool. London: RCN.

Gray, J.A.M. (2001) *Evidence-based Health Care: How to Make Policy and Management Decisions* (2nd edn). Edinburgh: Churchill Livingstone.

Gray, M.A. and Smith, L.N. (2000) 'The qualities of an effective mentor from the student nurse's perspective: Findings from a longitudinal qualitative study', *Journal of Advanced Nursing*, 32 (6): 1542–9.

Greenhalgh, T. (2006) *How to Read a Paper: The Basics of Evidence-Based Medicine*. Oxford: BMJ Books.

Griffiths, L., Worth, P., Scullard, Z. and Gilbert, D. (2010) 'Supporting disabled students in practice: A tripartite approach', *Nurse Education in Practice*, 10 (3): 132–7.

Guba, E.G. and Lincoln, Y.S. (1989) *Fourth Generation Evaluation*. London: Sage.

Guile, D. and Young, M. (1996) 'Further professional development and further education teachers: Setting a new agenda for work-based learning', in I. Woodward (ed.), *Continuing Professional Development: Issues in Design and Delivery*. London: Cassell.

Gutteridge, R. and Dobbins, K. (2010) 'Service user and carer involvement in learning and teaching: A faculty of health staff perspective', *Nurse Education Today*, 30 (6): 509–14.

Hall, K.M., Draper, R.J., Smith, L.K. and Bullough, Jr, R.V. (2008) 'More than a place to teach: Exploring the perceptions of the roles and responsibilities of mentor teachers', *Mentoring & Tutoring: Partnership in Learning*, 16 (3): 328–45.

Hallin, K. and Danielson, E. (2009) 'Being a personal preceptor for nursing students: Registered nurses' experiences before and after introduction of a preceptor model', *Journal of Advanced Nursing*, 65 (1): 161–74.

Handy, C. (1989) *Age of Unreason*. London: Business Books.

Hargreaves, J. (1996) 'Credit where credit's due: Work-based learning in professional practice', *Journal of Clinical Nursing*, 5 (2): 165–9.

Harrison, J., Dymoke, S. and Pell, T. (2006) 'Mentoring beginning teachers in secondary schools: An analysis of practice', *Teaching and Teacher Education*, 22 (8): 1055–67.

Harrison, S. (2005) 'Closing the poverty trap between study and work [Analysis]', *Nursing Standard*, 19 (40): 15–16.

Hawkins, P. and Shohet, R. (2006) *Supervision in the Helping Professions* (3rd edn). Milton Keynes: Open University Press.

Health Professions Council (HPC) (2006) *Your Guide to our Standards for Continuing Professional Education*. London: HPC.

Health Professions Council (HPC) (2008) *Standards of Proficiency – Operating Department Practitioners*. Available at: www.hpc-uk.org/publications/standards/index.asp?id=46. Accessed 4 January 2010.

Health Professions Council (HPC) (2009) *Standards of Education and Training Guidance*. Available at: www.hpc-uk.org/assets/documents/1000295FStandardsofeducationandtrainingguidance-fromSeptember2009.pdf. Accessed 4 January 2010.

Health Professions Council (2010) *About Registration – Professions*. Available at: www.hpc-uk.org/aboutregistration/professions/. Accessed 20 May 2010.

Hean, S., Clark, J.M., Adams, K., Humphris, D. and Lathlean, J. (2006) 'Being seen by others as we see ourselves: The congruence between the in-group and outgroup perceptions of health and social care students', *Learning in Health and Social Care*, 5 (1): 10–22.

Heirs, B. and Farrell, P. (1986) *The Professional Decision Thinker*. London: Sidgwick & Jackson.

Hemingway, P. and Brereton, N. (2009) *What is a Systematic Review?* Available at: www.medicine.ox.ac.uk/bandolier/painres/download/whatis/Syst-review.pdf. Accessed 30 July 2010.

Henderson, A., Twentyman, M., Heel, A. and Lloyd, B. (2006) 'Students' perception of the psychosocial clinical learning environment: An evaluation of placement models', *Nurse Education Today*, 26 (7): 564–71.

Henderson, A., Creedy, D., Boorman, R., Cooke, M. and Walker, R. (2010) 'Development and psychometric testing of the Clinical Learning Organisational Culture Survey (CLOCS)', *Nurse Education Today*, 30 (7): 598–602.

Heron, J. (1989) *Six Category Intervention Analysis: Human Potential Research Project* (2nd edn). Guildford: University of Surrey.

Higher Education Academy (2005) *Occasional Paper 6: Making Practice–Based Learning Work*. Available at: www.health.heacademy.ac.uk/publications/occasionalpaper/occp6. pdf. Accessed 7 May 2010.

Hinton, J. (2009) 'Mentorship: The experiences of a tutor in a pre-registration operating department practice education programme', *Journal of Perioperative Practice*, 19 (7): 221–4.

Holt, J., Coates, C., Cotterill, D., Eastburn, S., Laxton, J., Young, C. and Mistry, H. (2010) 'Identifying common competences in health and social care: An example of multi-institutional and inter-professional working', *Nurse Education Today*, 30 (3): 264–70.

Honey, P. and Mumford, A. (2000) *The Learning Styles Helper's Guide*. Maidenhead: Peter Honey.

Hughes, C. (1999) 'The dire in self-directed learning', *Adults Learning*, 11 (2): 7–9.

Hughes, L. and Marsh, T. (2006) *Planning for an Interprofessional Workforce: Creating an Interprofessional Workforce (CIPW) Programme*. Available at: www.dh.gov.uk/ Policy AndGuidance. Accessed 25 May 2006.

Hunt, J. (1981) 'Indicators of nursing practice: The use of nursing research findings', *Journal of Advanced Nursing*, 6 (3): 189–94.

Hunt, J. (1997) 'Towards evidence-based practice', *Nursing Management*, 4 (2): 14–17.

Hutchings, A. and Sanders, L. (2001) 'Developing a learning pathway for student nurses', *Nursing Standard*, 15 (40): 38–41.

Institute of Directors (2010) *Executive Coaching*. Available at: http://en.wikipedia.org/ wiki/Institute_of_Directors. Accessed 14 June 2010.

Institute of Healthcare Improvement (IHI) (2010) *Testing Changes*. Available at: www.ihi. org/IHI/Topics/Improvement/ImprovementMethods/HowToImprove/ testingchanges.htm. Accessed 1 June 2010.

Issakidis, C. and Andrews, G. (2006) 'Who treats whom? An application of the Pathways to Care model in Australia', *Australian & New Zealand Journal of Psychiatry*, 40 (1): 74–86.

James, S., D'Amore, A. and Thomas, T. (2011) 'Learning preferences of first year nursing and midwifery students: Utilising VARK', *Nurse Education Today*, 31, in press, doi: 10.1016/j.nedt.2010.08.008.

Jarvis, P. (1995) *Adult and Continuing Education*. London: Croom Helm.

Jarvis, P. and Gibson, S. (1997) *The Teacher Practitioner and Mentor* (2nd edn). Cheltenham: Stanley Thornes.

Jeffs, T. (2003) 'Quest for knowledge begins with a recognition of shared ignorance', *Adults Learning*, 14 (6): 28.

Johansson, U., Kaila, P., Ahlner-Elmqvist, M., Leksell, J. and Isoaho, H. (2010) 'Clinical learning environment, supervision and nurse teacher evaluation scale: Psychometric evaluation of the Swedish version', *Journal of Advanced Nursing*, 66 (9): 2085–93.

Joyce, B., Calhoun, E. and Hopkins, D. (2009) *Models of Learning: Tools for Teaching* (3rd edn). Maidenhead: Open University Press.

Kane, A. and Gooding, C. (2009) *Reasonable Adjustments Nursing and Midwifery – Literature Review*. Available at: www.nmc-uk.org/aDisplayDocument.aspx?DocumentID=5772. Accessed 5 May 2010.

Kendall-Raynor, P. (2007) 'Nurse cleared in supervision case is to face NMC', *Nursing Standard*, 21 (17): 9.

Kerry, T. and Mayes, A.S. (eds) (1995) *Issues in Mentoring*. London: Routledge/Open University.

Kirkpatrick, D. L. and Kirkpatrick, J. D. (2005) *Evaluating Training Programs: The Four Levels* (3rd edn). San Francisco, CA: Berrett-Koehler.

Knowles, M., Holton III, E.F. and Swanson, R.A. (1998) *The Adult Learner* (5th edn). Woburn, MA: Butterworth-Heinemann.

Koh, L. C. (2010) 'Academic staff perspectives of formative assessment in nurse education', *Nurse Education in Practice*, 10 (4): 205–9.

Kohler, W. (1925) 'The mentality of apes', in E. Smith, S. Nolen-Hoeksema and B. Fredrickson (eds) (2003), *Atkinson and Hilgard's Introduction to Psychology* (14th edn). London: Thomson/Wadsworth.

Kolb, D. (1984) *Experiential Learning: Experience as the Source of Learning and Development*. London: Prentice-Hall.

Kopp, P. (2001) 'Fit for practice – 6.1: What is evidence-based practice?', *Nursing Times*, 97 (22): 47–50.

Kouzes, M. and Posner, B.Z. (2007) *The Leadership Challenge* (4th edn). New York: Jossey-Bass.

Kramer, M. (1974) *Reality Shock: Why Nurses Leave Nursing*. St Louis, MO: Mosby.

Krathwohl, D.R. (2002) 'A revision of Bloom's *Taxonomy*: An overview', *Theory into Practice*, 41 (4): 212–18.

Krathwohl, D., Bloom, B. and Masia, B. (1999) *A Taxonomy of Educational Objectives: The Classification of Education Goals, Handbook 2: Affective Domain* (2nd edn). Harlow: Longman.

Lakasing, E. and Francis, H. (2005) 'The crisis in student mentorship', *Primary Health Care*, 15 (4): 40–1.

Lang, N. (1976) *Issues in Quality Assurance in Nursing: ANA Issues in Evaluative Research*. Kansas City, KS: American Nursing Association.

Lankshear, A. (1990) 'Failure to fail: The teacher's dilemma', *Nursing Standard*, 4 (20): 35–7.

Lewin, K. (1951) *Field Theory in Social Science*. London: Harper & Row.

Liefer, D. (2002) 'Do you have a plan?', *Nursing Standard*, 16 (41): 14–17.

Liefer, D. (2005) 'My practice: Government policy changes allowed an entrepreneurial nurse to pave the way for nurse-led general practices', *Nursing Standard*, 19 (22): 58.

Lindberg, J.B., Hunter, M.L. and Kruszewski, A.Z. (1998) *Introduction to Nursing: Concepts, Issues and Opportunities* (3rd edn). Philadelphia, PA: Lippincott.

Livneh, C. and Livneh, H. (1999) 'Continuing professional education among educators: Predictors of participation in learning activities', *Adult Education Quarterly*, 49 (2): 91–106.

Lloyd, N. (1999) 'BJTR and interdisciplinary practice: Moving forward', *British Journal of Therapy and Rehabilitation*, 6 (12): 573.

Lloyd-Jones, N., Hutchings, S. and Hobson, S.H. (2007) 'Interprofessional learning in practice for pre-registration health care: Interprofessional learning occurs in practice – Is it articulated or celebrated?', *Nurse Education in Practice*, 7 (1): 11–17.

Long, A., Kneafsey, R., Ryan, J. and Howard, J. (2001) *Exploring the Role and Contribution of the Nurse in the Multi-professional Rehabilitation Team (Research Highlights 45)*. Available at: www.nmc–uk.org/Documents/Archived%20Publications/ENB%20Archived%20Publications/ENB_ARCHIVED_PUBLICATION_Research%20Highlights%2045%20February%202001.PDF. Accessed 13 August 2010.

Luckhaupt, E., Chin, M.H., Mangione, C.M., Phillips, R.S., Bell, D., Leonard, A.C. and Tsevat, J. (2005) 'Mentorship in academic general internal medicine – results of a survey of mentors', *Journal of General Internal Medicine*, 20 (11): 1014–18.

Lunyk-Child, O.L., Crooks, D., Ellis, P.J., Ofosu, C., O'Mara, L. and Rideout, E. (2001) 'Self-directed learning: Faculty and student perceptions', *Journal of Nursing Education*, 40 (3): 116–23.

Madden, C. and Mitchell, V. (1993) *Professions, Standards and Competence: A Survey of Continuing Education for the Professions*. Bristol: Department for Continuing Education, University of Bristol.

Mallik, M. and McGowan, B. (2007) 'Issues in practice based learning in nursing in the United Kingdom and the Republic of Ireland: Results from a multi professional scoping exercise', *Nurse Education Today*, 27 (1): 52–9.

Marton, F., Hounsell, D. and Entwistle, N. (eds) (1997) *The Experience of Learning* (2nd edn). Edinburgh: Scottish Academic Press.

Maslow, A.H. (1987) *Motivation and Personality* (3rd edn). London: Harper & Row.

Maxwell, R.J. (1984) 'Quality assurance in health care', *British Medical Journal*, 288 (6428): 1470–2.

Mazhindu, G.N. (1990) 'Contract learning reconsidered: A critical examination of implications for application in nurse education', *Journal of Advanced Nursing*, 15 (1): 101–9.

McArthur, G.S. and Burns, I. (2008) 'An evaluation, at the 1-year stage, of a 3-year project to introduce practice education facilitators to NHS Tayside and Fife', *Nurse Education Today*, 8 (3): 149–55.

McCarthy, B. and Murphy, S. (2008) 'Assessing undergraduate nursing students in clinical practice: Do preceptors use assessment strategies?', *Nurse Education Today*, 28 (3): 301–13.

McCaughan, D., Thompson, C., Cullum, N., Sheldon, T.A. and Thompson, D.R. (2002) 'Acute care: Nurses' perceptions of barriers to using research information in clinical decision-making', *Journal of Advanced Nursing*, 39 (1): 46–60.

McCormack, B., Manley, K., Kitson, A., Titchen, A. and Harvey, G. (1999) 'Towards practice development – A vision in reality or a reality without vision?', *Journal of Nursing Management*, 7 (5): 255–64.

McGill, I. and Beatty, L. (1998) 'Continuing professional development', in C.M. Downie and P. Basford (eds), *Teaching and Assessing in Clinical Practice*. London: University of Greenwich.

McGivney, V. (2003) *Adult Learning Pathways: Through Routes or Cul-de-sac*. Leicester: NIACE.

McGregor, D. (1987) *The Human Side of Enterprise*. London: Penguin.

McKenna, H.P. (1995) 'Dissemination and application of mental health nursing research', *British Journal of Nursing*, 4 (21): 1257–63.

McKimm, J., Jollie, C. and Hatter, M. (2007) *Mentoring: Theory and Practice*. Available at: www.faculty.londondeanery.ac.uk/e-learning/explore-further/e-learning/feedback/files/Mentoring_Theory_and_Practice.pdf. Accessed 29 July 2010.

McNicholl, M.P., Dunne, K., Garvey, A., Sharkey, R. and Bradley, A. (2006) 'Using the Liverpool care pathway for a dying patient', *Nursing Standard*, 20 (38): 46–50.

Megginson, D. and Clutterbuck, D. (2005) *Techniques for Coaching and Mentoring*. Oxford: Elsevier.

Megginson, D., Clutterbuck, D., Garvey, B., Stokes, P. and Garrett-Harris, R. (2006) *Mentoring in Action: A Practical Guide*. London: Kogan Page.

Mezirow, J. (1983) 'A critical theory of adult learning and education', in M. Tight (ed.), *Adult Learning and Education*. London: Croom Helm.

Mikkelsen Kyrkjebø, J. and Hage, I. (2005) 'What we know and what they do: Nursing students' experiences of improvement knowledge in clinical practice', *Nurse Education Today*, 25 (3): 167–75.

Miller, C., Ross, N. and Freeman, M. (1999) *The Role of Collaborative/Shared Learning in Pre-and Post-Registration Education in Nursing, Midwifery and Health Visiting (Research Highlights 39)*. Available at: www.nmc-uk.org/Documents/Archived%20Publications/ ENB%20Archived%20Publications/ENB_ARCHIVED_PUBLICATION_ Research%20Highlights%2039%20July%201999.PDF. Accessed 8 October 2010.

Morrison, S., Boohan, M., Moutray, M. and Jenkins, J. (2004) 'Developing pre-qualification interprofessional education', *Nurse Education in Practice*, 4 (1): 20–9.

Mott MacDonald (2009) *Quality Assurance Handbook – September 2009*. Available at: www.nmc.mottmac.com/infoprogproviders/. Accessed 2 May 2010.

Mulholland, J., Scammell, J., Turnock, C. and Gregg, B. (2006) *Making Practice-based Learning Work: Final Report*. Northumbria: Northumbria University.

National Committee of Inquiry into Higher Education (NCIHE) (1997) *Higher Education in the Learning Society (The Dearing Report)*. Norwich: HMSO.

Neary, M. (2000a) *Teaching, Assessing and Evaluation for Clinical Competence*. Cheltenham: Stanley Thornes.

Neary, M. (2000b) 'Responsive assessment of clinical competence (Part 1)', *Nursing Standard*, 15 (9): 34–6.

Newton, J.M., Billett, S. and Ockerby, C.M. (2009) 'Journeying through clinical placements – An examination of six student cases', *Nurse Education Today*, 29 (6): 630–4.

Newton, J.M., Jolly, B.C., Ockerby, C.M. and Cross, W.M. (2010) 'Clinical Learning Environment Inventory: Factor analysis', *Journal of Advanced Nursing*, 66 (6): 1371–81.

NHS Evidence (2010) *Sources of Information*. Available at: www.evidence.nhs.uk/ aboutus/Pages/SelectingInformationSources.aspx. Accessed 29 July 2010.

NHS Institute for Innovation and Improvement (NHS III) (2010) *Transforming Good Ideas into Workable Solutions for the NHS*. Available at: www.institute.nhs.uk/. Accessed 22 September 2010.

Nicklin, P. and Kenworthy, N. (eds) (2000) *Teaching and Assessing in Nursing Practice: An Experiential Approach* (3rd edn). London: Baillière Tindall.

Norman, I.J., Watson, R., Murrells, T., Calman, L. and Redfern, S. (2002) 'The validity and reliability of methods to assess the competence to practise of pre-registration nursing and midwifery students', *International Journal of Nursing Studies*, 39 (2): 123–244.

Northcott, N. (1989) 'Planning the transition from student to staff nurse', *Senior Nurse*, 9 (7): 27–8.

Nursing and Midwifery Council (NMC) (2004a) *Standards of Proficiency for Pre-Registration Nursing Education*. London: NMC.

Nursing and Midwifery Council (NMC) (2004b) *Reporting Unfitness to Practise: A Guide for Employers and Managers.* London: NMC.

Nursing and Midwifery Council (NMC) (2004c) *Standards of Proficiency for Specialist Community Public Health Nurses.* London: NMC.

Nursing and Midwifery Council (NMC) (2005a) *NMC Consultation on Proposals Arising from a Review of Fitness for Practice at the Point of Registration.* London: NMC.

Nursing and Midwifery Council (NMC) (2005b) *NMC Approved Standard for Practice Teachers. NMC Circular 39/2005.* Available at: www.nmc-uk.org/Documents/Circulars/2005%20circulars/NMC%20circular%2039_2005.pdf. Accessed 31 August 2010.

Nursing and Midwifery Council (NMC) (2006a) *Preceptorship Guidelines. NMC Circular 21/2006.* Available at: www.nmc-uk.org. Accessed 18 April 2010.

Nursing and Midwifery Council (NMC) (2006b) *Responses to the NMC Consultation on Proposals Arising from a Review of Fitness for Practice at the Point of Registration. Final Report.* London: NMC.

Nursing and Midwifery Council (NMC) (2007a) *Ensuring Continuity of Practice Assessment through the Ongoing Achievement Record. NMC Circular 33/2007.* Available at: www.nmc-uk.org/Documents/Circulars/2007%20circulars/NMC%20circular%2033_2007.pdf. Accessed 10 August 2010.

Nursing and Midwifery Council (NMC) (2007b) *Sign-off Status and Preceptorship for Practice Teacher Students. NMC Circular 27/2007.* Available at: www.nmc-uk.org/aDisplayDocument.aspx?DocumentID=3261. Accessed 5 May 2010.

Nursing and Midwifery Council (NMC) (2007c) *Introduction of Essential Skills Clusters for Pre-registration Nursing programmes. NMC Circular 07/2007* (first published 20 March 2007, updated 4 September 2008). Available at: www.nmc-uk.org/Documents/Circulars/2007%20circulars/NMC%20circular%2007_2007.pdf. Accessed 13 August 2010.

Nursing and Midwifery Council (NMC) (2008a) *A Standard to Support Learning and Assessment in Practice.* London: NMC.

Nursing and Midwifery Council (2008b) *The Code: Standards of Conduct, Performance and Ethics for Nurses and Midwives.* London: NMC.

Nursing and Midwifery Council (NMC) (2008c) *The PREP Handbook.* Available at: www.nmc-uk.org/Documents/Standards/nmcPrepHandbook.pdf. Accessed 20 May 2010.

Nursing and Midwifery Council (NMC) (2009a) 'Revalidation', *NMC News,* 30 (November): 5. Available at: www.nmc-uk.org/aDisplayDocument.aspx?DocumentID=6791. Accessed 15 March 2010.

Nursing and Midwifery Council (NMC) (2009b) *NMC Review of Pre-registration Nursing Education Bulletin* (3 April). Available at: www.nmc-uk.org/aDisplayDocument.aspx?DocumentID=5945. Accessed 18 April 2010.

Nursing and Midwifery Council (NMC) (2009c) *Record Keeping: Guidance for Nurses and Midwives.* Available at:www.nmc-uk.org/aDisplayDocument.aspx?DocumentID=6269. Accessed 12 May 2010.

Nursing and Midwifery Council (NMC) (2009d) *Additional Information to Support Implementation of NMC Standards to Support Learning and Assessment in Practice.* Available at: www.nmc-uk.org/Documents/Standards/nmcAdditionalinformaionForSuppor LearningAndAssessmentInPractice2008.pdf. Accessed 7 June 2010.

Nursing and Midwifery Council (NMC) (2009e) *Standards for Pre-registration Midwifery Education.* Available at:www.nmc-uk.org/aDisplayDocument.aspx?DocumentID=5700. Accessed 20 May 2010.

Nursing and Midwifery Council (NMC) (2010a) *Standards for Pre-registration Nursing Education*. Available at: http://standards.nmc-uk.org/PreRegNursing/statutory/background/Pages/Introduction.aspx. Accessed 18 September 2010.

Nursing and Midwifery Council (NMC) (2010b) *Sign-off Mentor Criteria. NMC Circular 05/2010*.Available at: www.nmc-uk.org/aDisplayDocument.aspx?DocumentID=7807. Accessed 9 April 2010.

O'Driscoll, M.F., Allan, H.T. and Smith, P.A. (2010) 'Still looking for leadership – Who is responsible for student nurses' learning in practice?', *Nurse Education Today*, 30 (3): 212–17.

Office of Public Sector Information (OPSI) (2001) *Special Educational Needs and Disability Act 2001*. Available at: www.opsi.gov.uk/acts/acts2001/ukpga_20010010_en_1. Accessed 19 March 2010.

Office of Public Sector Information (2005) *Disability Discrimination Act 2005*. Available at: www.england-legislation.hmso.gov.uk/acts/acts2005/ukpga_20050013_en_1. Accessed 19 March 2010.

Open University (2001) *Assessing Practice in Nursing and Midwifery – K320 Workbook 3*. Milton Keynes: Open University Press.

Orton, H. (1981) 'Ward learning climate and student nurse response', *Nursing Times*, 77 (17): 65–8.

Orton, H.D., Prowse, J. and Millen, C. (1993) *Charting the Way to Excellence (Ward Learning Climate Project)*. Sheffield: Sheffield Hallam University.

Overill, S. (1998) 'A practical guide to care pathways', *Journal of Integrated Care*, 2: 93–8.

Page, S. (2001) 'Demystifying practice development', *Nursing Times*, 97 (22): 36–7.

Paice, E., Heard, S. and Moss, F. (2002) 'How important are role models in making good doctors', *British Medical Journal*, 325 (7366): 707–10.

Palfreyman, S., Tod, A. and Doyle, J. (2003) 'Comparing evidence-based practice of nurses and physiotherapists', *British Journal of Nursing*, 12 (4): 246–53.

Pedler, M., Burgoyne, J. and Boydell, T. (1997) *The Learning Company – A Strategy for Sustainable Development*. London: McGraw-Hill.

Peters, R.S. (1966) *Ethics and Education*. London: George Allen & Unwin.

Peters, R.S. (1973) *The Philosophy of Education (Oxford Readings in Philosophy)*. Oxford: Oxford University Press.

Phillips, T., Schostak, J. and Tyler, J. (2000) *Practice and Assessment: An Evaluation of the Assessment of Practice at Diploma, and Degree and Post-graduate Level in Pre- and Post-registration Nursing and Midwifery Education (Research Highlight 43)*. Available at: www.nmc-uk.org/Publications-/Circulars/Circulars-2007/Search?access=p&entqr=0&output=xml_no_dtd&sort=date%3AD%3AL%3Ad1&ie=UTF-8&client=NMC_Live&q=Practice+and+Assessment+in+Nursing+and+Midwifery%3A+Doing+it+for+Real&filter=0&ud=1&site=NMC_Live&oe=UTF-8&proxystylesheet=NMC_Live&ip=10.15.0.100&start=0. Accessed 13 August 2010.

Piaget, J. (1962) 'The stages of intellectual development of the child', in I. Roth (ed.), *Introduction to Psychology*. Milton Keynes: LEA/Open University.

Pirrie, A., Wilson, V., Harden, R.M. and Elsegood, J. (1998) 'Multiprofessional Education: Part two – promoting cohesive practice in healthcare (AMEE Guide No. 12)', *Medical Teacher*, 20 (5): 409–16.

Polanyi, M. (1958) *Personal Knowledge*. London: Routledge.

Pollard, C. and Hibbert, C. (2004) 'Expanding student learning using patient pathways', *Nursing Standard*, 19 (2): 40–3.

Price, A. and Price, B. (2009) 'Role modelling practice with students on clinical placements', *Nursing Standard*, 24 (11): 51–6.

Price, B. (2007) 'Practice-based assessment: Strategies for mentors', *Nursing Standard*, 21 (36): 49–56.

Price, B. (2010) 'Disseminating best practice through teaching', *Nursing Standard*, 24 (27): 35–41.

Proctor, B. (2001) 'Training for the supervision alliance: Attitude, skills and intention', in J. Cutcliffe, T. Butterworth and B. Proctor (eds), *Fundamental Themes in Clinical Supervision*. London: Routledge.

Quality Assurance Agency for Higher Education (QAA) (2001) *Guidelines for HE Progress Files*. Available at: www.qaa.ac.uk/academicinfrastructure/progressFiles/guidelines/progfile2001.pdf. Accessed 23 August 2010.

Quality Assurance Agency for Higher Education (QAA) (2006) *Code of Practice for the Assurance of Academic Quality and Standards in Higher Education. Section 6: Assessment of Students*. Available at: www.qaa.ac.uk/academicinfrastructure/codeOfPractice/section6/COP_AOS.pdf. Accessed 24 August 2010.

Quality Assurance Agency for Higher Education (QAA) (2007) *Code of Practice for the Assurance of Academic Quality and Standards in Higher Education. Section 9: Work-based and Placement Learning*. Available at: www.qaa.ac.uk/academicinfrastructure/codeofpractice/section9/placementlearning.pdf. Accessed 12 July 2010.

Quality Assurance Agency for Higher Education (QAA) (2008) *The Framework for Higher Education Qualifications in England, Wales and Northern Ireland*. Available at: www.qaa.ac.uk/academicinfrastructure/FHEQ/EWNI08/FHEQ08.pdf. Accessed 20 May 2010.

Quality Assurance Agency for Higher Education (QAA) (2009) *Handbook for Institutional Audit: England and Northern Ireland*. Available at: www.qaa.ac.uk/reviews/institutional Audit/handbook2009/InstitutionalAuditHandbook2009.pdf. Accessed 1 June 2010.

Quality Assurance Agency for Higher Education (QAA) (2010) *Code of Practice for the Assurance of Academic Quality and Standards in Higher Education. Section 3: Disabled Students*. Available at: www.qaa.ac.uk/academicinfrastructure/codeofpractice/section3/section3disabilities2010.pdf. Accessed 3 July 2010.

Quinn, F.M. and Hughes, S.J. (2007) *Quinn's Principles and Practice of Nurse Education* (5th edn). Cheltenham: Nelson Thornes.

Race, P. (2010) *Making Learning Happen – A Guide for Post-compulsory Education* (2nd edn). London: SAGE Publications.

Ramsden, P. (2003) *Learning to Teach in Higher Education* (2nd edn). London: RoutledgeFalmer.

Rattray, J.E., Paul, F. and Tully, V. (2006) 'Partnership working between a higher education institution and NHS Trusts: Developing an acute and critical care module', *Nursing in Critical Care*, 11 (3): 111–17.

Redfern, S. (1998) 'Evaluation: Drawing comparisons or achieving consensus?', *NTresearch*, 3 (6): 464–74.

Reeves, S. and Pryce, A. (1998) 'Emerging themes: An exploratory research project of an interprofessional education module for medical, dental and nursing students', *Nurse Education Today*, 18 (7): 534–41.

Roberts, P., Priest, H. and Bromage, C. (2001) 'Selecting and utilising data sources to evaluate health care education', *Nurse Researcher*, 8 (3): 15–29.

Rogers, A. and Horrocks, H. (2010) *Teaching Adults* (4th edn). Berkshire: McGraw-Hill Education.

Rogers, C. (1983) *Freedom to Learn in the 80s.* Columbus: Charles Merrill.

Rogers, C. and Freiberg, H.J. (1994) *Freedom to Learn* (3rd edn). Upper Saddle River, NJ: Pearson Education.

Rogers, E. and Shoemaker, F. (1971) *Communication of Innovations: A Cross-cultural Report* (2nd edn). New York: Free Press.

Rolfe, G. (1999) 'Insufficient evidence: The problems of evidence-based nursing', *Nurse Education Today*, 19 (6): 433–42.

Rotem, A. and Hart, G. (1995) 'The clinical learning environment: Nurses' perceptions of professional development in clinical settings', *Nurse Education Today*, 15 (1): 3–10.

Rowntree, D. (1987) *Assessing Students: How Shall We Know Them?* London: Kogan Page.

Royal College of Nursing (RCN) (1996) *The Royal College of Nursing Clinical Effectiveness Initiative: A Strategic Framework.* London: RCN.

Royal College of Nursing (RCN) (2002) *Helping Students Get the Best from Their Practice Placements (A Royal College of Nursing Toolkit).* London: RCN.

Royal College of Nursing (RCN) (2003) *Quality Education for Quality Care: A Position Statement for Nursing Education.* London: RCN.

Royal College of Nursing (RCN) (2004) *The Future Nurse: Evidence of the Impact of Registered Nurses.* London: RCN.

Royal College of Nursing (RCN) (2005) *Maxi Nurses: Nurses Working in Advanced and Extended Roles Promoting and Developing Patient-centred Healthcare.* London: RCN.

Royal College of Nursing (RCN) (2006) *Practice Development.* London: RCN.

Royal College of Nursing (RCN) (2007) *Guidance for Mentors of Nursing Students and Midwives: An RCN Toolkit.* London: RCN.

Rycroft-Malone, J., Harvey, G., Kitson, A., McCormack, B., Seers, K. and Titchen, A. (2002) 'Getting evidence into practice', *Nursing Standard*, 16 (37): 38–43.

Sackett, D.L., Rosenburg, W., Gray, J.M., Haynes, R.B. and Richardson, S.W. (1996) 'Evidence-based medicine: What it is and what it isn't', *BMJ*, 312 (7023): 71–2.

Sackett, D.L., Strauss, S.E., Richardson, S.W., Rosenburg, W. and Haynes, R.B. (2000) *Evidence-based Medicine: How to Practice and Teach EBM* (2nd edn). Edinburgh: Churchill Livingstone.

Salmon, D. and Jones, M. (2001) 'Shaping the interprofessional agenda: A study examining qualified nurses' perceptions of learning with each other', *Nurse Education Today*, 21 (1): 18–25.

Satterly, D. (1981) *Assessment in Schools: Theory and Practice in Education.* Oxford: Blackwell Science.

Scammell, B. (1990) *Communication Skills.* Basingstoke: Macmillan.

Scheler, M. (1980) *Problems of Sociology of Knowledge.* London: Routledge & Kegan Paul.

Schon, D. (1995) *The Reflective Practitioner: How Professionals Think in Action.* Aldershot: Arena.

Scottish Government (2010) *Flying Start NHS.* Available at: www.flyingstart.scot.nhs.uk/index.htm. Accessed 12 January 2010.

Scullion, P. (2002) 'Effective dissemination strategies', *Nurse Researcher: Qualitative Approaches*, 10 (1): 65–7.

Scullion, P. A. (2010) 'Models of disability: Their influence in nursing and potential role in challenging discrimination', *Journal of Advanced Nursing*, 66 (3): 697–707.

Shardlow, S. and Doel, M. (1996) *Practice Learning and Teaching*. London: British Association of Social Workers/Macmillan.

Sharp, M. (2000) 'The assessment of incompetence: Practice teachers' support needs when working with failing DipSW students', *Journal of Practice Teaching*, 2 (3): 5–18.

Simpson, J. and Weiner, E. (1989) *The Oxford English Dictionary* (2nd edn). Oxford: Oxford University Press.

Sines, D., Harris, D., Firth, J. and Boden, L. (2006) 'Applied leadership: Ensuring fitness for practice', *Nursing Management*, 13 (8): 28–31.

Skinner, B.F. (1971) *Beyond Freedom and Dignity*. New York: Alfred Knopf.

Sleep, J. and Clark, E. (1999) 'Weighing up the evidence: The contribution of critical literature reviews to the development of practice', *NTresearch*, 4 (1): 306–13.

Smith, J. and Rudd, C. (2010) 'Implementing the productive ward management programme', *Nursing Standard*, 24 (31): 45–8.

Spouse, J. (2001a) 'Bridging theory and practice in the supervisory relationship: A socio-cultural perspective', *Journal of Advanced Nursing*, 33 (4): 512–22.

Spouse, J. (2001b) 'Work-based learning in healthcare environments', *Nurse Education in Practice*, 1 (1): 12–18.

Steinaker, N.W. and Bell, M.R. (1979) *The Experiential Learning: A New Approach to Teaching and Learning*. New York: Academic Press.

Stevens, D. (2003) 'The practice educator in specialist community practice', *Journal of Community Nursing*, 17 (2): 30–1.

Stewart, S. and Carpenter, C. (2009) 'Electronic mentoring: An innovative approach to providing clinical support', *International Journal of Therapy and Rehabilitation*, 16 (4): 199–206.

Stickley, T., Stacey, G., Pollock, K., Smith, A., Betinis, J. and Fairbank, S. (2010) 'The practice assessment of student nurses by people who use mental health services', *Nurse Education Today*, 30 (1): 20–5.

Stuart, C.C. (2007) *Assessment, Supervision and Support in Clinical Practice* (2nd edn). Edinburgh: Churchill Livingstone.

Sullivan, E.J. and Decker, P.J. (2009) *Effective Leadership and Management in Nursing* (7th edn). Upper Saddle River, NJ: Pearson Education.

Tee, S.R., Owens, K., Plowright, S., Ramnath, P., Rourke, S., James, C. and Bayliss, J. (2010) 'Being reasonable: Supporting disabled nursing students in practice', *Nurse Education in Practice*, 10 (4): 216–21.

Thiroux, J. and Krasemann, K. (2007) *Ethics, Theory and Practice* (9th edn). Upper Saddle River, NJ: Pearson/Prentice-Hall.

Thomas, L. (2005) 'An inspiration to all', *Nursing Standard*, 19 (24): 27.

Thompson, C. (1998) 'Testing our intuition', *Nursing Standard*, 12 (27): 18.

Thompson, C., McCaughan, D., Cullum, N., Sheldon, T. and Raynor, P. (2002) 'The value of research in clinical decision-making', *Nursing Times*, 98 (42): 30–4.

Titchen, A. (2003) 'The practice development diamond'. Paper presented at the 2003 *International Nursing Research Conference*, London.

UNISON (2006) *Learning the Hard Way*. London: UNISON.

United Kingdom Central Council for Nursing, Midwifery and Health Visiting (UKCC) (1999) *Fitness for Practice.* Available at: www.nmc-uk.org/Documents/Archived%20 Publications/UKCC%20Archived%20Publications/Fitness%20for%20Practice%20 and%20Purpose%20The%20UKCC%20Commission%20for%20Nursing%20 and%20Midwifery%20Education%20Summary%20September%201999. PD. Accessed 18 July 2010.

United Kingdom Central Council for Nursing, Midwifery and Health Visiting (2000) *The Scope of Professional Practice: A Study of Its Implementation.* Available at: www. nmc-uk.org/Documents/Archived%20Publications/UKCC%20Archived%20 Publications/Perceptions%20of%20the%20Scope%20of%20Professional%20 Practice%20January%202000.PDF. Accessed 18 July 2010.

Unsworth, J. (2000) 'Practice development: A concept analysis', *Journal of Nursing Management,* 8 (6): 317–26.

van Eps, M., Cooke, M., Creedy, D. and Walker, R. (2006) 'Student evaluations of a year-long mentorship program: A quality improvement initiative', *Nurse Education Today,* 26 (6): 519–24.

van Wijngaarden, J.D.H., Dirks, M., Dippel, D.W.J., Minkman, M. and Niessen, L.W. (2006) 'Towards effective and efficient care pathways: Thrombolysis in acute ischaemic stroke' *Qjm,* 99 (4): 267–72.

Viney, R. and McKimm, J. (2010) 'Mentoring', *British Journal of Hospital Medicine,* 71 (2): 106–9.

Waddington, K. and Marsh, L. (1998) 'Work-based learning in a multigrade, multiskilled group: An action research perspective', *Managing Clinical Nursing,* 2 (4): 101–4.

Wallace, M. (1999) *Lifelong Learning: PREP in Action.* Edinburgh: Churchill Livingstone.

Walsh, M. and Ford, P. (1989) *Nursing Rituals, Research and Rational Actions.* Oxford: Heinemann Nursing.

Ward, C. and McCormack, B. (2000) 'Creating an adult learning culture through practice development', *Nurse Education Today,* 20 (4): 259–66.

Ward, L., Fenton, K. and Maher, L. (2010) 'The high impact actions for nursing and midwifery 3: Staying safe, preventing falls', *Nursing Times,* 106 (29): 12–13.

Waskett, C. (2010) 'Clinical supervision using the 4S model 1: Considering the structure and setting it up', *Nursing Times,* 106 (16): 12–14.

Waters, D., Clarke, M., Ingall, A.H. and Dean-Jones, M. (2003) 'Evaluation of a pilot mentoring programme for nurse managers', *Journal of Advanced Nursing,* 42 (5): 516–26.

Watkins, K. and Marsick, V. (1992) 'Building the learning organisation: A new role for human resource developers', *Studies in Continuing Education,* 14 (2): 115–29.

Watson, J.B. (1978) 'The great psychologists: From Aristotle to Freud', in E. Smith, S. Nolen-Hoeksema and B. Fredrickson (eds) (2003), *Atkinson and Hilgard's Introduction to Psychology* (14th edn). London: Thomson/Wadsworth.

White, E., Davies, S., Twinn, S. and Rilet, E. (1993) *A Detailed Study of the Relationship between Teaching, Support, Supervision, and Role Modelling for Students in Clinical Areas within the Context of Project 2000 Courses (Research Highlight 3).* Available at: www. nmc-uk.org/Documents/Archived%20Publications/ENB%20Archived%20 Publications/ENB_ARCHIVED_PUBLICATION_researchHighlights3December1 993%5b1%5d.PDF. Accessed 8 October 2010.

White, J. (2007) 'Supporting nursing students with dyslexia in clinical practice', *Nursing Standard,* 21 (19): 35–42.

Wilkinson, J. (1999) 'A practical guide to assessing nursing students in clinical practice', *British Journal of Nursing*, 8 (4): 218–22.

Williamson, G. (2009) 'Student support on placement: The student experience and staff perceptions of the implementation of placement development team', *The 2009 RCN International Nursing Research Conference – Book of Abstracts* (section 9.1.3): 107.

Wilson, V., Pirrie, A. and Finnigan, J. (1998) 'Encouraging learning: A study of continuing professional development in health care', *Health Bulletin*, 56 (3): 667–74.

Wood, S. (2005) 'The experiences of a group of pre-registration mental health nursing students', *Nurse Education Today*, 25 (3): 189–96.

Wright, S. (1990) *Building and Using a Model of Nursing*. London: Edward Arnold.

Wright, S.M. and Carrese, J.A. (2002) 'Excellence in role modelling: Insight and perspectives from the pros', *Canadian Medical Association Journal*, 167 (6): 638–43.

Young, P., Moore, E., Griffiths, G., Raine, R., Stewart, R., Cownie, M. and Frutos-Perez, M. (2010) 'Help is just a text away: The use of short message service texting to provide an additional means of support for health care students during practice placements', *Nurse Education Today*, 30 (2): 118–23.

# Index